Awaken the
Diet Within

Awaken the Diet Within

From Overweight Mom to Beauty Queen—My Nine Steps to Successful Weight Loss

JULIA GRIGGS HAVEY

WARNER BOOKS

An AOL Time Warner Company

Neither this diet nor any other diet program should be followed without first consulting a health care professional. If you have any special conditions requiring attention, you should consult with your health care professional regularly regarding possible modification of the program contained in this book.

Copyright © 2002 by Julia Griggs Havey
All rights reserved.

Portions of this book were previously published in *Awaken the Diet Within* and *Take-Control Recipes*, both published in 1998 by The Health and Wellness Institute.

"Self-Improvement through Self-Motivation" is a trademark owned by The Health and Wellness Institute.

Warner Books, Inc., 1271 Avenue of the Americas, New York, NY 10020

Visit our Web site at www.twbookmark.com.

 An AOL Time Warner Company

Printed in the United States of America

Originally published in hardcover by Warner Books, Inc.
First Trade Printing: January 2004
10 9 8 7 6 5 4 3 2 1

The Library of Congress has cataloged the hardcover edition as follows:

Havey, Julia Griggs.
    Awaken the diet within : from overweight to looking great—if I can do it, so can you / Julia Griggs Havey.
        p. cm.
    ISBN 0-446-53016-6
    1. Weight loss. I. Title.

    RM222.2 .H315 2003
    613.2—dc21   2002024998
ISBN: 0-446-69122-4 (pbk.)

Book design by Giorgetta Bell McRee
Cover photo by Suzy Gorman

Dedicated to the memory of Bill Maritz, leader in the field of motivation, and a civic leader, father, friend, and mentor. Thank you for believing in me. You gave your time, listened, offered advice, and masterfully condensed my message into the simple phrase "Self-Improvement through Self-Motivation." Your time on this earth was cut short, but your thoughts, insight, vision, and goodwill live on and will continue to help improve the lives of others.

Acknowledgments

I would like to thank you for purchasing this book and for believing that together we can get you firmly on the path of Self-Improvement through Self-Motivation. I want you to read this as though we are sitting across the table from each other, sharing a cup of coffee (or a glass of water) and just talking as friends. Thousands of people are realizing their dreams and goals as a result of the journey you are about to start. It is a joy and a privilege to be their guide, and now yours, along this path. It will be paved with challenges, hurdles, rejoicing, and smiles, but most important it is a path of true and permanent change.

This book is the compilation of years of work, learning, and growth. It would never have been possible without the support and effort of so many people. Thanking them all would require another book. There are a few, however, who must be mentioned.

First, Linda Konner, my agent extraordinaire, who took a risk on an "unknown" and proved that success takes just "one more try." Her efforts fulfilled the first of my three wishes: having a publisher!

Thanks to Diana Baroni, my editor at Warner Books, who is wise beyond her years. Her vision and foresight allowed her to see that this book had the ability to change people's lives. Her editorial talent and love of books have helped to make this into what I dreamed it could be. Diana, thanks for fulfilling my second wish: to allow this book to reach as many people as possible and teach them they can realize their dreams and goals simply by awakening the power they have within themselves. I thank everyone at Warner Books for working so hard on this book, especially Molly Chehak, Penina Sacks, and Flamur Tonuzi.

To my family, you fulfilled my third and final wish: to live happily ever after. To my beautiful and talented "Diva" daughter, Taylor (Warner Music, are you listening?), and my outrageously funny and athletic son, Clark (future West Point cadet), thanks for being such great children and for being so patient in allowing me to follow my dream. To my fabulous husband, Patrick, I thank God every day for putting you in our lives. You are the best husband, partner, friend, and father in the world. You always challenge me to be the best I can be. Your belief in me is the wind in my sail. This book would not be a reality if not for you. You not only complete me but improve me. I love you so much. The best is yet to come.

To my father, you are the most honorable man I have ever met. The creed you learned at West Point, "Duty, Honor, and Country," has been passed on to me. I am lucky to know you and am proud to be your daughter. I love you.

To my family, sisters, brothers-in-law and sisters-in-law, nieces, nephews, and friends, you all have been wonderfully supportive of me, and I can never thank you enough. Thanks for never giving up on me and for always being there to catch me when I fall.

To Rosie and John, the best in-laws anyone could ask for. They have spent their lives helping others and have set a wonderful example for us to follow. They lead by their example of compassion and commitment to strong family values.

Thanks must also be given to my dear friend and editor at eDiets.com, John McGran. He believes in me and my message and helped me reach millions of "dieters" through my "Take It Off w/Julia" and Master Motivator articles. Many thanks, "Boss"!

I would also like to thank God for the blessings He has put in my life. I have not always been open to the lessons that were meant for me to learn, and I am thankful that He never quit trying to teach me. Please give me the faith to continue to follow and serve You as You see fit for me!

Contents

Guide for Starting Over

The following is a prayer that I keep in my wallet. As I was starting my journey, it gave me strength; today it renews that strength. These are words of great wisdom, regardless of your faith.

May I have the courage to begin again—
may I be ready to overlook the
difficulties, to overcome the obstacles
and to stay open to the moment
as best I can.

May I be patient enough to know
it takes time to start over,
and wise enough to ask for help
from friends and family
when I need it.

As I look to the future,
may I reflect on the past
and remember the lessons
it's taught me.

And, Lord, may I always remember
to look to You
for strength and guidance.

*Used with the permission of Abbey Press.

Introduction:
Awakening My Diet Within

It was a typical day, making breakfast for the kids, packing lunches, and rushing to get everyone ready so I could make it to the office on time. I would drop Taylor at school, swing Clark to the baby-sitter's, make a quick stop at the bread store to get my bran muffin and diet Pepsi. I was on yet another diet.

On my way to work I ran into traffic, which gave me a few minutes more to listen to the morning DJ's jokes and enjoy my "alone" time. Loneliness was something I was familiar with. Even with two young children constantly clamoring for attention, one can feel very alone without a husband and father around regularly. That was what I had: a husband who wasn't around much. He worked long hours as a laborer—hard, physically demanding work. After work, he and his co-workers would often gather for a few beers to unwind. This ritual kept him out late many nights. When he did make it home, the kids were usually in bed. Good thing, as it kept them from hearing us bicker about where he had been and why he wasn't home more often. The time we did have together was spent arguing about the amount of time we didn't spend together.

Other than the arguments, I thought things were fine in our relationship. I accepted it as love when he referred to me teasingly as "the prettiest fat lady he'd ever seen" or when he would "moo" at me as I was heading toward the cookie jar. He liked to tease. He had a good sense of humor; it had been one of the traits that drew me to him. We had been in love once. Coincidentally, I was thinner then and we didn't have kids and money worries. But now my way of dealing with my life was to eat my worries away. There seemed to be nothing a pastry couldn't fix.

On the way home from work, I stopped by Baskin-Robbins for my daily dose of "diet" Espresso and Creme "light" ice cream. My spirits were lifted and my thoughts of wanting to lose weight were far away. Besides, I was eating something good for me—it was "light"! Food and my weight controlled my every thought and action back then. I had myself convinced that if I kept up the bran muffin, ice cream, and pasta with cheese diet and made it to step class twice a week, I would be svelte again in no time. Not only that, but my marriage would also be improved, and we would spend more time together as a family. It was going to be Ward and June Cleaver perfect. I believed that all of my problems were the fault of my weight. I was tired of watching all the other families at the park looking so happy—dads pushing their children on the swings, smiling at the mom, who looked perfect wearing her little white shorts and cute top, complete with a dainty pair of sandals and bright red toenails. It wasn't fair that my kids only had "fat" me waving to them from the park bench. As I ate a hamburger, sitting there in my oversized shift and leggings with toenails that were badly in need of a pedicure showing through my beat-up old flip-flops, I wished that I too could be like the "thin" moms. I would never venture into the play structure with them for fear that I would get stuck or, worse, that someone would comment on my weight. So I sat on the bench watching everyone else have fun, convinced that "tomorrow" my life would change.

Once I arrived home, I shuffled through the day's mail. A letter addressed to me with no return address caught my eye. In the moment it took for me to tear open the envelope and read its two simple sentences, my life was forever changed. The letter revealed something I should have seen long ago. The clues were there for me to see all along, but I just never wanted to put the pieces together. The message slapped me in the face as I read it over and over again:

Your husband is having an affair with ———— and it has been going on for over two years. Follow him next time he goes to ————.

It actually named her and told me where to follow him. I was devastated!

I had no idea what to do next. I figured it must be some cruel joke by someone who didn't like me. After all, two weeks earlier my husband had promised me that he "would never have an affair" as had our friend's husband. He stressed that we would always be together. The baby was only a year old; how could he have been with someone for over two years? It just didn't make sense. But then again it explained so much. No matter, I just did not want to believe it was true. Maybe he wasn't the play-with-the-kids-in-the-park kind of family man I dreamed of, but he did call me every day and told me that he loved me. He believed in me and he was my friend. I just didn't know what to think.

Despite the recent decline of romance in our life, I still loved my husband very much. Why else would I be so upset? I thought of all the positive things in our relationship—the funny jokes, the backgammon games, the trips we had taken. Then it dawned on me that all of these memories were from a very long time ago. There wasn't much recent fun or romance. There wasn't much to convince me that this letter wasn't true. I remember clearly coming up with what I thought was the solution: "I will diet and lose weight and then we will be happy again."

I paged him at his job site, saying that it was a family emergency. I needed to hear him tell me that he loved me, that this was a cruel prank, and that life would go on as normal. To my relief, he did in fact reassure me. He was very angry and said he would find out who was trying to hurt me with these lies. As he hung up the phone, my heart sank. Despite his adamant denial, I couldn't stop crying.

I called my family and closest girlfriends. They had no doubt that the letter was true and they felt that no matter how painful, it was better to know the truth than to continue living a lie. My family and friends urged me to use the situation to start to change all that had been wrong with my life for far too long. In many ways, they were glad this had happened. They had witnessed my husband's odd behavior at our wedding, watched me show up alone at numerous couples' get-togethers, and had heard of his antics long enough to convince them that I deserved more out of life. The problem was that this was all I felt worthy of—after all, I was fat.

My unhappiness had manifested itself in my thighs, and was very hard to hide from the world. The consensus among my girlfriends was that I overate to hide from the problems in my marriage. I had two small children and I didn't want to raise them alone. Being married, no matter how unhappily, suited me just fine. They didn't understand that the self-assured Julia they used to know would have left her husband long before this recent revelation. My friends and their husbands had long ago lost any respect for my husband.

It was my fault that everything was so haywire in my life. I thought I was the one who had gotten out of control and that I didn't deserve to be happy. My friends and family didn't understand what had happened to the self-assured Julia they used to know.

The Julia I had become was scared of divorce, and scared of an unsure future. More than anything, I was scared that things would never improve for me—that I was and always would be an obese, matronly, frumpy, unhappy, and crabby person. At thirty years of age, this is how I had come to view myself. I feared things worsening; I feared becoming a statistic: a woman with children dumped for a younger babe, forced to sell my house, live in a trailer, and survive on one income and child support, with little money for any extras. I felt that most women don't end up better after a divorce, so I didn't want to be the recipient of one. I loved my home and had always dreamed of my children being able to grow up living in the same house, attend the same school, and have the same friends through high school. I was the product of numerous moves and divorced parents, and I didn't want that for my children. I had convinced myself that an absentee dad was better than none at all. At least that way we had two incomes, money for bikes, movies, pizza parties—the perfect suburban childhood. And of course my mind began to race with thoughts like: "I am fat—who would want to date me?" I had been called fat for so long that it had become a *personality trait,* rather than just a *physical condition.* What a mess my life had become. I didn't know what to do next other than take a trip to the bakery, for there was nothing a napoleon or two couldn't soothe.

When my husband arrived home that evening, I would like to tell you I kept my composure and was cool and collected, but that would be untrue. I fell apart and I begged him to stay, assuring him that I would lose weight and we would be happy again. He laughed off my concerns and feelings and told me not to be so upset He said something like, "There is no one else—we'll always be married." He buried his head farther in the sand, and for the first time in years I began to pull mine out.

One of the first steps I took was to sign us up for marriage counseling. I found a wonderful counselor and his wife who help couples rebuild their relationships. I started going, in hopes that it would help us have the close and loving marriage I dreamed of—the kind we never had but that I hoped we would grow into. My husband reluctantly joined me. He felt there was no need for counseling and stuck firmly to his insistence that there was no "other woman." I became the lunatic who just wouldn't "drop it."

I continued my scheduled counseling sessions even when he eventually dropped out. I kept learning things about myself that I had never known, and I rediscovered things long forgotten. Each week I felt stronger and more secure with who I was. Interestingly enough, I was losing weight, too! I had thought that losing weight was going to solve all my problems, but it just didn't seem to be working as I had dreamed. Counseling helped me to make sense out of my situation, discover who I was, and get on the path to realizing who I wanted to be. I began to realize that you can only change yourself, not others. You must strive to be the best person that you can be, and only then can you positively impact the world around you. That's a lot different than trying to change those around you, thinking the problem lies with them.

The final straw came one morning when my baby son was sick. He had a temperature of 103 degrees, and I took the day off to stay home with him. My husband left for work at his usual 5:30 A.M. departure time for his 8:00 A.M. start time.

As I drove to the drugstore to get my son some medicine, I couldn't stop thinking about the affair. I found myself making a quick U-turn and heading for the love shack—the address given on the anonymous note. I had to see for myself if in fact my husband actually spent his mornings there. You guessed it: The pickup truck was in the driveway. I literally drove into her front yard and at the top of my lungs started yelling for him to come out. I shouted the nature of his visit, enlightening all of her neighbors and embarrassing the heck out of myself. I was not proud of my behavior, nor of his. Eventually the adulterer sulked out of his mistress's house carrying his work boots and lunch box. The jig was up. The denials were over. He had been caught red-handed by the "fat lunatic," as my husband described me. He couldn't lie his way out of it this time. In his opinion, I was the one at fault for daring to follow him and not trusting him.

That was the final day of my marriage, although in reality it had been over many years before. I was no longer willing to subject myself to that kind of humiliation. The pain and, at the same time, the release I felt that day were like nothing I had ever experienced. I was scared, yet exhilarated. Mad, yet relieved. I was also at least forty pounds lighter at that point and was confident that, with time, I would get my life and my body back in order, for myself and for the children.

Later that day I threw everything my husband owned onto the front porch. Nothing has ever felt so freeing. As he watched his belongings being tossed out, he pleaded with me to let him stay, saying that he loved us and didn't want to leave. He didn't have the ability to tell me the truth even then. He loved the children and really didn't want to leave them, but he sure didn't want to be my husband. He didn't want to hurt me any more than I had already been hurt, but he didn't realize that each day we lived together only made my life worse. We didn't have, nor would we ever have, the kind of marriage I had dreamed of as a little girl. It was not my dream to wash a man's clothes and care for his children but let him have a girlfriend on the side. Life with him was keeping me from finding a loving relationship, while he had found his. It was time to move on. We were both sad to end our chance at the perfect family, and I understood that it wasn't his intention to hurt me; he was trying to find something he felt was missing in his life. Although his actions were inexcusable, I can't say my patterns of behavior over the years helped the relationship.

For over two and a half years I had felt like a prison warden, not a wife, as I dared to question my husband's whereabouts and actions. My self-esteem had been torn down bit by bit, my heart ripped out more and more each day. My thighs grew bigger and bigger out of my eating for companionship. Food had been my solace.

But now I was gaining confidence each day, and with that confidence came rationality. I have never looked back on that period of my life with regret, but rather as something to learn from. I knew that no matter how hard the road ahead became, I would survive. I had to—there was no other acceptable choice.

That was my awakening. My rock bottom. Your story may be similar to mine, or if you are lucky you have not yet lost something precious to you. Hopefully, joy hasn't been stolen from you because of your weight, or you have noticed the things you may be robbing yourself of. I used to look back on those months, and years, and wonder whether my husband quit loving me because I got fat or whether *I* quit loving me and got fat. The latter would have made it impossible for anyone to love me—not because I was overweight, but because I didn't love myself.

My weight loss began as my attempt to save my marriage. I believed that my weight was to blame for all of my problems. It is important to note that the fear of ending my marriage was a big stick motivating me to change. Not everything can be saved if you wait too long to take action. It is important to note that when it comes to making major changes in our lives, we need a big stick to motivate us—and it helps even more to have a big carrot!

Perhaps reading of my plight will urge you into action before something sacred in your life is lost. As I write of that painful period in my life, I do it knowing that there are many of you out there who are tolerating less than respectful treatment from others and, most important, from yourselves. You are accepting it because of low self-esteem. Think of your life and what is at risk: your health, your relationships, your career—the list goes on and on. All of it can be improved when you take back control of your life.

I do not want readers to think I blame anyone but myself for the events that happened in my life. In order to realize true changes, you must get to the point where you understand and believe that you and you alone are in control of and responsible for your own actions. A bad marriage did not make me overweight—eating too much food did.

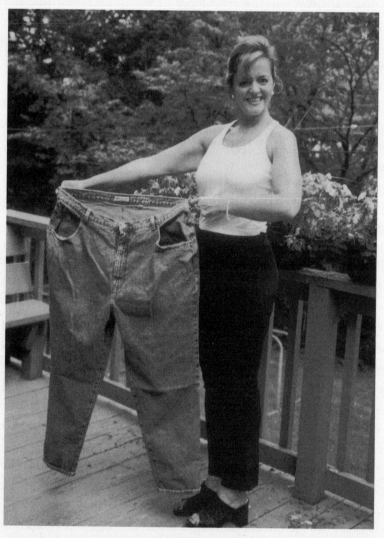

The new me, 130 pounds lighter.

If what happened to *me* can teach *you* one lesson, I hope that it is not to let food consume you, especially to the point where you quit cherishing all of the gifts of life. Your new motto should be: *I consume food, but I don't let it consume me.* I don't know if my marriage could have been a happy one had I not gotten overweight, or if we would have grown closer rather than apart. I do not regret the path I've traveled because it has made me who I am today, and I have learned from it. It has taught me never to take life, myself, or those I love for granted ever again. I have also learned that being overweight has many more negative effects in your life than just ruining your health. It *can* rob you of a full and rewarding life by keeping you from your true potential as a person.

I continued to work on self-improvement, even though my marriage was over. For the first time in my life, my weight loss was for me, for my health, for my happiness To make what would be a very long story short, I lost 130 pounds over the course of 15 months. That averages out to 8 pounds a month, 2 pounds a week, and mere ounces a day. While those numbers may sound impressive, they pale in comparison to the other changes brought about in my life through self-improvement.

I kept custody of my children, kept the house, and created a stable life for myself. I started dating and soon fell in love with a wonderful man. After a whirlwind courtship, we ran off to Las Vegas and got married. I had an intense desire to shout my story from the highest mountaintop, letting the world know how happy I was and how losing weight enabled me to change my life. I wrote my story and sent it to *Women's World* magazine. They sent a reporter and photographer to my house and ran a full-page article on

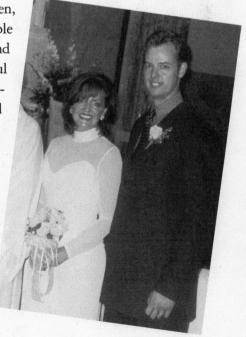

me. As if that weren't enough of a thrill, the *Sally Jesse Raphael Show* then called and invited me to share my story on national television. The *National Enquirer* called and asked to run a piece on me. My first response was, "As long as it doesn't read 'Woman with 3 Eyes Lost 130 Pounds'—sure!" I had my fifteen minutes of tabloid fame. We were flooded with inquiries from women asking me questions, applauding my transformation, and asking me how they too could do what I did.

My new husband, Patrick, suggested that I start by telling them *why* I changed my life and then give them my method and secrets so

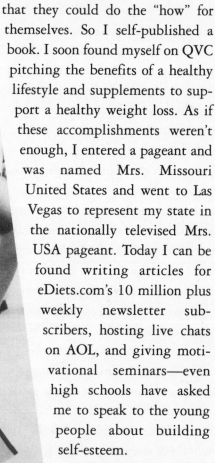

that they could do the "how" for themselves. So I self-published a book. I soon found myself on QVC pitching the benefits of a healthy lifestyle and supplements to support a healthy weight loss. As if these accomplishments weren't enough, I entered a pageant and was named Mrs. Missouri United States and went to Las Vegas to represent my state in the nationally televised Mrs. USA pageant. Today I can be found writing articles for eDiets.com's 10 million plus weekly newsletter subscribers, hosting live chats on AOL, and giving motivational seminars—even high schools have asked me to speak to the young people about building self-esteem.

I know that you are now thinking you mistakenly bought a fairytale novel, but you have not. What

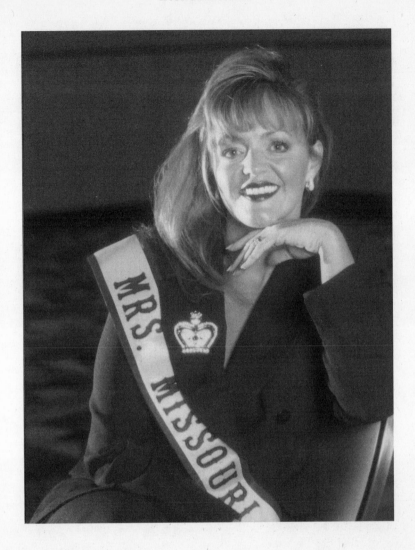

you have bought is a book that will supply you with all of the tools you need to chart your own successful weight-loss journey. In this book I am going to help you tap into your "diet" within, help you identify all of the reasons why you want to change and what those changes will mean for your life. I lay out for you a gradual slope of positive actions that will allow you to realize success upon success and, in doing so, rebuild shattered self-esteem. You will learn the way to exercise, to eat, and to think more positively about yourself. You will be motivated to—and learn how to—awaken your diet within!

PART I

—————

My Story

From the Beginning

It took me until age thirty-five to realize and embrace the fact that we are *not* our bodies. Your body is the vehicle that houses who you are, that which makes you uniquely you—your soul, your being. Identical twins may have bodies that look the same, but their souls and personalities are completely different and individual. Realize that your body does not define who you are now, nor will it when you are thinner. This concept is similar to the misconception that simply having more money will make people happy when, in reality, if they're not happy without money, chances are they won't be happy with it.

My obsession with my weight and body image began long before I became heavy. In fact, I had spent most of my thirty-plus years obsessed with my body. Throughout my life, I'd find myself thinking things like "I'm too fat, my thighs are too big, my chest is too small." I measured my self-worth by how others viewed my body and how they treated me. I sought my self-esteem via others' image of me based upon the appearance of my body, rather than through *my* image of myself—spiritually and emotionally—the person inside who really mattered.

My father enjoys telling the story of my first brush with overeating. After I was born, my mother required a few more days in the hospital to recoup from an infection. Since Dad had managed to raise two other babies without incident, they felt it was safe to send me home alone with him. He marveled in his skill at caring for me. I was a perfect baby, for a girl. He was 0 for 3 at attempts for a son. I was healthy, and could I eat! I was certainly thriving. My weight had nearly doubled in the week following my birth. It wasn't until my mother arrived home and pointed out to him that you have to dilute the formula that he realized I was merely bloated and about to explode.

I wasn't a particularly fat kid, but I wasn't a skinny one either. Regardless of size, I remember other children teasing me and calling me "Griggs Pigs." I vividly remember being crushed when a saleslady announced that I couldn't fit into a size 6X any longer. That moment might be what triggered my size obsession. A 6X was tiny, petite, cute kid clothes! I didn't want to wear the plus-size big-kid clothes. I think I just didn't want to grow up. But continue to grow I did. As children can be cruel, I doubt that any of them realized how badly their school-yard pranks hurt. It just seems to be human nature to make fun of people who are different.

The name calling and my continuous growth didn't curb my appetite. When my friends and I discovered my mother's stash of premade desserts in the freezer in the carport, we devoured them. After all, who would miss a few—dozen! I will never forget my mother's reaction when she found them missing. That negative reinforcement should have been enough to curb my closet eating, but it wasn't.

Once my junk-food source had been cut off, I began sneaking to the store on my bike to buy Pop-Tarts with my friends and gorge on them before we got home. That was the beginning of my unhealthy eating habits: I was a self-taught closet eater. It was the family mystery: Why did Julia keep getting bigger?

At thirteen, I had a lot on my plate, both figuratively and literally. My parents were divorcing and my sisters were going off to college. For a while it was just my dad, Nana, and myself. Talk about bad eating habits. We ate either the outrageously good, though very fattening, southern-fried soul food my nana's helper made us, or my dad's "roast in a bag" special. I often stuck with the Pop-Tarts. That's when I developed my habit for skipping meals and eating only sweets.

In the next few years, my dad retired from the United States Air Force and we bought a house in St. Louis. Finally, I thought, we had a permanent home. I would be able to have friends I could get to know well and not have to say good-bye to in a few months. A school where I could get to be part of the cliques—no more of these schools by the base where the locals have all known each other their whole lives and aren't about to let military brats into their circles. I was really looking forward to this.

My weight wasn't bad then; I felt like a normal teenage girl. I wore a size ten or twelve, and by my definition I wasn't fat or even chubby. Things went well for me at my new school. I had a boyfriend the first year. I met seven girls in my Spanish class. We were known as the Big 8—eight girls, each one crazier than the next!

My friends and I all shared the same appetites, as well, and we could easily evacuate a refrigerator after school, sometimes without the formality of silverware. However, the world can be an unfair place. After all, they never seemed to gain weight. That appeared to be *my* job.

Although I was relatively thin at the time, or so I thought, a few boys in school would often tease me by calling me "Namu the killer whale" and "Buffalo butt." How bullies are able to locate your weak point and then exploit it is beyond me, but there are those who are so good at it they make it an art form.

A girl with high self-esteem would have realized that these pimple-faced boys were merely looking for attention from one in the more popular group, a point that I, of course, could recognize only with the wisdom of a grown woman. As a young girl, it drove me to the Diet Center for an entire summer, slimming down to a practically anorexic 110 pounds—at five feet, eight inches tall, that's a bit extreme. My willpower was intense that summer; the girls and I all went to an outdoor concert and I drank only my diet soda with lime while they imbibed in a few (root?) beers. I got so thin that summer that my boyfriend du jour's father bought a candy bar and made me eat it. I can look back now, with wisdom, and see so clearly that I made stupid decisions out of an attempt to gain acceptance. I wasn't secure with who I was. I needed to hear from others that they thought I was great because I didn't think very highly of myself.

How well I remember the craziness of weight obsession in my teen years: the unhealthy diets, the desperate thoughts, and the strange rationalizations. There is not a diet out there I haven't tried. Once, out of pure desperation, I offered a friend $500 to drive me to a hospital emergency-department entrance and have her chop off my rear end. Then the doctors would take me into the hospital and sew me up. Sure, I'd be horribly scarred, I thought, but at least I'd be thinner. (You've never been that desperate?) Another time, a friend and I jogged to the all-night bakery and ate a dozen cream-filled doughnuts. I guess we figured we could eat as much as we wanted since we had jogged a few blocks. Let me tell you, getting back was a lot harder than getting there!

You can't name a fad diet I haven't tried. I'm sure that now you'll believe that I once bought "miracle weight-loss pants" from an ad in the back of a magazine. You know those ads: "Amazing! Drop 20 Pounds and a Dozen Inches in Two Days!" Maybe you purchased the pants as well? The ad promised inches off my waist by the very next morning. I waited weeks for my package to arrive, eating all I could in the duration, assured that the svelte body I sought was "in the mail." The package came and I ran upstairs with it, tearing it open along the way.

In preparation for the magical transformation, I ran back downstairs to get the vacuum cleaner, then back upstairs to pull on the miracle pants, which were made of something that resembled a plastic trash bag. I attached them to the vacuum as instructed and commenced running in place. I guess the idea was that I would vacuum out the fat from my body. Things went great for about

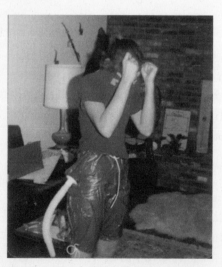

thirty seconds. Then, in all the excitement, the unthinkable happened. The rear end of the pants split wide open. I was released from the compression seal and, thus, a complete "blowout"! I was devastated. My dreams of a "Playmate figure" were shattered. Not only had I not lost inches, but my eating spree while waiting for the miracle to arrive in the mail left me with more pounds and inches to contend with. I don't think my family ever took any of my dieting seriously from that moment on.

In my senior year of high school, all I talked about was becoming an ADPi, a sorority my mother had joined in college. She was the campus beauty queen and a teen Miss Florida—an Elizabeth Taylor double and an actual descendant of Spanish royalty. On her side of the family we are related to the original first family of Florida, back to Ponce de León and all the conquistador history. I have a photo from *Town & Country* magazine of my mother and grandmother posing with the reigning royal family member. If only America still used formal titles so I could go by the title Contessa Julia!

I didn't know my mother very well; I have seen her only a few times since my parents divorced. I do remember her, though, as the outwardly perfect southern woman, very graceful and charming to others. I felt that joining her old sorority would somehow make us closer. Growing up without her all those years, I wanted more of a connection to her. I never told anyone why this was so important to me; everyone thought I just wanted the social fun of belonging to a sorority, but to me it meant more—a lot more. I would share something with my mother that was a huge part of her life. Joining that sorority and being part of that group was all I wanted out of college. I guess I thought that would make up for the mother I didn't have.

When I began college, I was much too immature and unprepared to be on my own. I had no clue what I wanted to be when I grew up, or even if I wanted to grow up. My ignorance during those days stretched so far as to question my friend Betsy, who knew that she wanted to become an engineer. I thought, Why in the world would she want to operate a train? My grades in high school reflected my don't-give-a-darn attitude at the time, and therefore the sorority system that I so desperately wanted to be part of turned up its nose at me—Ouch! They pushed my dreams aside without so much as a chance to prove myself worthy. I had blown my chances without even knowing it.

I was miserable at college. I felt like everyone belonged to something except me. I really tried to fit into the college scene, but it never seemed to work for me. I became very depressed and plunged farther into my eating disorders. I even dabbled with bulimia.

My dad insisted that I pull myself together, that I tell my professors I was sorry and would work hard to make up the work I had missed. But it wasn't as if I had the confidence to walk up to a professor and admit erring. That was my whole problem. I lacked any belief in myself or my abilities, academically or personally. I allowed not getting into a sorority to eat me up inside. I felt like a big loser.

At one point, though, I did manage to confront my philosophy teacher. He was understanding; perhaps he knew that my self-esteem was very low. He convinced me to stick with school and try. He would rank as one of those wonderful people whom I have been lucky enough to encounter along the way who really cared about me and tried to get me to see that I was more than what I gave myself credit for.

After a few more years of the same, my dad eventually tired of my academic-probation status and suggested I take a break—maybe to become a stewardess. So I left school in hopes that change would do me good. I was accepted for the stewardess position, and it gave me great happiness to have been accepted—I finally belonged to an elite group. There was the weight requirement, though, and as time went on I noticed (as did my boss) that I was always on the high end, literally, of the acceptable weight limit. Much like at the air force bases, when I was the boss's daughter, I caught a lot of flack now. My dad ran the airport in St. Louis and this was the largest airline in the city. It was always "She's *his* kid," or "Wonder how *you* got the job?" So much for fitting in and being accepted. But that didn't keep me from having a great time. I really loved the job and I was good at it as well. To me, it was like hosting a dinner party every night: It was my job to make sure that all passengers not only got to their destinations safely, but also had a great time getting there. I was beginning to realize my strengths: I was social, not academic. I loved working first class on the long flights—the airline's service was very elaborate then (and so was the food).

The layovers as a stewardess (of course, "flight attendant" now) were a blast. We went sight-seeing in different cities and participated in a lot of social activities. One such layover in Hawaii, coupled with too much sun, made for a very long flight home. I remember passengers feeling so sorry for my sunburned and blistered legs that they took out their aloe and rubbed me down.

My more professional crew members didn't enjoy my style. I thought that they believed I shouldn't be having fun because I was bordering the weight limit, and that I should take this matter seriously. I missed the point. It wasn't my weight that they took issue with; it was my lack of maturity and decorum. I thought then that everything revolved around my weight.

The variety of restaurants across the country made for great eating. My years in college had conditioned me for eating to feel good. Too good, in my case—I started filling out. Much to my embarrassment, my male boss summoned me to his office so that he could weigh me, asking, "Hop on the scale, Miss Griggs."

Weighing in was a serious matter. If I was too heavy, I could be grounded or put on weight check. For years I struggled to control my eating and maintain my weight. Laxatives became a food group for me. I didn't think I looked overweight back then, and I had only the airline's rules to keep me in check.

Out at the bars one night during an airline strike, I met a union man who kept giving me a hard time about crossing the picket line and not supporting my union. He was handsome, in a burly sort of way, and I suggested he try to change my mind over dinner. Laughing to my friends, I joked, "Watch me fall for this one!" You guessed it: I married him. We had a great time together. My weight started creeping up after one year of marriage—I was at about 160 pounds, compared to 135 when we married.

In hindsight, I am not sure how in love I really was. I think that even my decision to marry was mostly a matter of acceptance. My husband told me on our first date that his "wife and children would always come first." That sounded great to me.

To my relief, I became pregnant just at the time the airline would have required me to lose fifteen pounds. I now had a license to eat. I remember thinking, "Hey, I can gain all the weight I want now and the airline can't do a thing about it." Talk about cutting off your nose to spite your face—or, in my case, to stuff my face!

And stuff it I did. I was eating for two, wasn't I? Two pastries, two sundaes; I took full advantage of the situation. I wonder if any of my first-class passengers noticed that their dessert offerings were skimpier on my flights than on others. And, although I gained sixty-five pounds during my pregnancy, I didn't feel fat; I felt amazing. I thought I was the cutest pregnant lady ever and dismissed the weight gain, convinced that the reason I had gotten so big was that the next NFL superstar was in my womb. I guess I didn't realize that it isn't physically possible to "carry" in the rear end—my biggest part. I had a tiny baby girl—six pounds, three ounces. Hardly big enough to justify sixty-five pounds of weight gain. So, along with my beautiful baby I brought home fifty-plus pounds from the hospital.

Being fat rarely entered my mind. I basked in the joys of motherhood. I loved it! And since I was breast-feeding, of course I needed extra nutrition to produce enough milk. Bring on the buffet. Needless to say, I wasn't one of those women who are able to wear their pre-maternity clothes within weeks of delivery.

I gave up my flying career after accepting an early-retirement offer. Good thing I didn't return to my job as a stewardess, because I never could have squeezed into my uniform. I enjoyed my time off with my baby Taylor and I had actually started to trim down. My ten-year high school reunion was that summer and I starved myself until I could wear this super little red dress. Even though I was bigger than I was when I was in high school, I thought I looked great.

I loved being a stay-at-home mom. I could have done it forever if we could have afforded it. Instead, I entered the nine-to-five, sit-on-your-butt-all-day business world. My thighs and rear end thrived in this environment. I nibbled on snacks all day. My only exercise was walking to the snack machine—little wonder that I kept getting bigger. My reunion weight-loss diet was thrown out the window, and I added a few more pounds. Despite my weight gain, things were looking up. I had found my calling at this job: sales. I had finally found a job where my gift of gab didn't get me in trouble, but actually made me successful.

I am a born salesperson. I really loved what I was doing for a living. It was a great feeling being good at my job and enjoying it.

The only problem for me was that my desk job was so sedentary. As a flight attendant I moved around the airplane all day and walked a lot in the cities I stayed in. I was never a jogger or an exercise type of person, but at least I was moving. The most physical activity I got then was taking the baby to the park—I would walk from the car to the bench and sit down. Sometimes I even pushed her on the swings. It never even dawned on me to consider adding exercise to my routine. My husband didn't get any exercise; it just wasn't part of our lifestyle. We went out to eat for our socializing. We didn't even do that as often as we used to. I wasn't into the party lifestyle anymore, and I longed to be at home with my daughter when I wasn't working. Given my lack of movement and my increased appetite, I gradually kept getting bigger—it happens so slowly that you hardly notice the pounds creeping up. It starts with a belt that is too tight here, an old pair of jeans that you can't zip up there. The new clothes I bought were more comfortable a size or two bigger. Before I knew it, all of my clothes had become the new baggy look. Eventually they seemed to have shrunk and then it was back to the tight look again. I really thought that the problem wasn't me, that they didn't make clothes like they used to. I certainly never set out to become obese. It just happened—one bite at a time.

Going Downhill

I don't believe anyone likes being overweight. I am aware of the various "fat acceptance" organizations and I just can't buy into them now—and I didn't when I was obese, either. Even if a person were truly happy being severely overweight, it is still unhealthy. Being overweight doesn't mean you are a bad person, or stupid or lazy. It is merely something that happens. The good news is that it is also something that can "un-happen." Being overweight is either something you have been for your entire life and know no other way, or, as with me, something that sneaked up on you. I got in a rut, and eating filled a void in my life. I worked full time, I had a baby to care for, bills that never seemed to be paid, and a marriage that didn't provide any companionship or romance. At the time, I knew of no reasons to want to be thin. My husband was more interested in going out with his friends and being with them than he was in being intimate with me, and that suited me just fine. He was never around for that or much of anything else. I was a single mother with two incomes, and a married woman with no husband. My daughter couldn't have cared less if I was getting fatter, and it didn't affect my job performance.

I thought my life was a relatively happy one. I attempted many times to lose weight. I bought every diet book available and listened to the experts. After two years of being on a continuous diet, I still had not lost any weight. In fact I was bigger. Desperate and frustrated, I concocted yet another of my great ideas. I tried to recruit my very thin friend Mary to wear a bikini and carry a sign that said AFTER. I, too, would be in a bikini, but with a BEFORE sign. Together we would stand on a busy street corner soliciting drivers for donations to my liposuction fund. I really thought it would work!

How is it that, with all these great ideas and energy, weight loss never worked for me? A woman I met at a pool party mentioned that she owned an aerobics studio and she thought I was "too pretty to carry around all that extra weight." Why do so many good-intentioned people say such things? She offered her help if I wanted it. Help with what? Getting a partner to share my life with? I thought to myself, "Help me be more understanding of my husband and his lifestyle?" After all, was she implying that I was fat? She must be blind! I had on my new gold-trimmed swimsuit, with a towel draped ever so carefully to camouflage my thighs. No one could see that I was fat. I was Jane Mansfield–like, Marilyn Monroe–ish, but not *overweight*. I had myself convinced that I was happy with how I looked.

For the next day or so, I thought about what the woman at the party had said, and after my initial rage wore off I decided to exercise at her aerobics studio. I attended classes three or four times a week, dying inside each time I noticed one of the hunk bodybuilder guys in the gym checking out the women in class—the skinny women in spandex. I prayed they wouldn't notice me (how could they not), at least not until I lost some weight. I sincerely wanted to become just like the other women in the class: thin and healthy. I did what they were doing. I came to class, I danced around, and I sweated. I was doing everything they were doing, although I don't know if they drove by the bakery after class to refuel like I did.

The aerobics teacher soon gave me a printout of a diet she recommended: the typical three meals a day, snacks thrown in, lots of veggies, fruit, and a lot of brown rice. It was the usual seven-day-a-week plan, every meal laid out for you to follow. "Too rigid and too much food for me," I thought. I looked at that diet and thought it would make me gain weight. It called for more food in a meal than I ate all day. Sure, it didn't include ice cream, but it was still too much food, with too strict a regimen.

That diet-and-exercise regimen didn't last long. Soon I had stopped exercising (I was convinced the laughter from the gym had to be the hard-bodied guys laughing at me, the obese woman dancing and jig-gling) and I was overeating again. The diet only gave me more ex-cuses to avoid the changes I didn't want to face. Besides, I had a good reason this time: There were too many meals in her plan. I knew what I needed to do. I had to begin eating only a bran muffin for breakfast and a salad the rest of the day. (One of several problems with that diet, of course, is that the bran muffin, while sounding like a healthy breakfast item, actually has twenty-five grams of fat.) From one ex-treme to the other I went. I'm sure you've been there, with frustra-tion causing you to quit and succumb to cookies and ice cream, as I did.

I tried a few more traditional diets as well. Jenny Craig didn't work for me. I spent weeks of my time and hundreds of dollars buying all of the prepackaged food and eating it as directed. I thought that it tasted okay, and I made myself eat it—and a little extra here and there (the food was low cal so a bit more couldn't hurt, right?). I went to the behavior-modification classes; I cheated and then I quit. It wasn't for me. Nutri/System was next. Their food left me ten pounds heav-ier and hundreds of dollars poorer. I think I believed that if I spent money—a lot of money—on a particular system I would feel obli-gated to stick with it. I thought that money spent would equal weight lost, not that my efforts should have anything to do with it. Eventually, after numerous such diets with no results, I resigned my-self to "fatdom."

One day I asked myself, "Julia, you've failed at every diet you ever tried—what are you going to do?" My answer: "I'm going to Disney World!" I took Taylor there for some fun and a break from the stress of dieting—well, to get away from work, too. After getting home from the trip, I took our film to be developed. Seeing the few photos of me, I went back to feeling depressed and started another diet.

I really just wasn't ready to take charge of my life. I was attempting to surrender myself to these diet plans and let them work for me rather than work for *my own* success. By this time, I had lost all credibility with everyone who knew me. They were sick of hearing me go on and on about my desire to be thin, meanwhile watching me eat a pastry or gorge on whatever food someone had brought to the office to share.

*Looking back, I'm sure I could
have been one of the characters—
I was as big as this one!!*

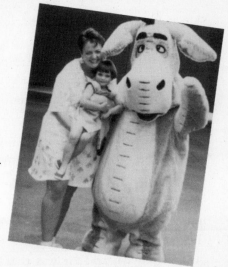

While the desire was there, I expected someone or something else
to do the work for me.

I refused to try on clothes at
stores for fear that I'd see my rear
end in one of those three-way mir-
rors—a sight that would depress me for days. I started
buying my clothes from mail-order catalogs. If no one saw me buy a
size-twenty-four pair of pants or the XX shirts, they wouldn't know
I wore that size, right? I really believed that as long as my clothes
were flowing dresses and baggy T-shirts people wouldn't notice how
big I was getting. For parties and holidays I always bought a new outfit and accessories; I thought this was great camouflage.

At that time in my life, I really thought I was trying to eat right.
I would watch in disbelief the amounts of junk food a large woman
(definition: anyone bigger than I was) at my office ate. One large
woman at my job would have a bag of cookies, chips, candy, and more
open on her desk and graze from them all day long. I wasn't doing
this, so I must have been eating right.

I would have "light" ice cream, good fresh bread with real butter,
huge salad-bar lunches, bakery goods—not the packaged junk food
the others ate. Why wasn't I losing weight?

My weight wasn't the only thing on a constant roller coaster. My
mood, attitude, and work-production level all were tied to my
weight. I hated the scale because it would dictate my mood. If the
scale indicated I had gained a few pounds, my mood and morale were
shot for the day—maybe even the week. I had no energy, no motivation, and no willpower. I lived to eat and hated myself for it. I was
negative and in a bad mood about everyone and everything in my life.

It was always the other guy's fault when something went wrong, never mine.

Does this sound familiar to you? Do you find yourself living the same self-defeating cycle? You get yourself totally motivated to lose the weight. You go to the extent and the expense of getting a gym membership or buying yet another piece of exercise equipment. Maybe a new book by an expert caught your eye: "the protein this" or "buster that." You went to the grocery store, loaded up on all the special foods your new and final diet insisted were the best and only way to eat, assured that this time you are going to do it. The first morning of the new diet, you wake up and you eat the half grapefruit and the two eggs. You don't combine carbos with proteins, or fruits with proteins, or whatever it was that the expert assured you was right. Later that day you even manage to say no to the doughnuts at the office. "Ha! Look at all those fools eating doughnuts," you think. You'll show them. You will be thinner than all of them soon! At the end of that long and self-sacrificing day, as you cook dinner for your family, your tuna awaits. You nibble on the kids' chicken and just a bite of the mashed potatoes. Just a little won't hurt you because you were so good today, right!? You can't deny yourself everything. One bite becomes several, and before long the tuna can wait for tomorrow or, even worse, you eat it too, so as to stay on track with your program. You'll be better tomorrow. Been there, done that—more times than I care to mention!

I was sick of dieting. It just didn't work. The diet experts couldn't be wrong; therefore the problem must be *me*. Feeling as if I no longer had a life to live, I plodded through an existence where, each day, mentally I was "eating" myself up. I would become anxious about meals—every meal—thinking about food more than about any other aspect of my life. Food consumed me, rather than me consuming it. I spent my day asking myself: "Did I eat too much? How can I still be hungry after eating all my lunch? Why did I overeat again—I can hardly move!" Decisions about food made me anxious, and if I made a "good" decision—to eat a healthy low-cal food or a small portion—I was preoccupied with how hungry I was and how unsatisfied it made me feel. If I made a "bad" decision I felt guilty, hated myself, and continually beat myself up about it the rest of the day. Every time I went on a diet I thought constantly about food, how much I could eat and when, even more so than when I wasn't dieting. By ten o'clock in the morning I was already stressing out about what to eat for lunch.

The only real joy I had during these years was coming home to my precious little girl: She didn't care if her mama was fat. She loved me for me. She was my approval, my acceptance of who I was. Watching her grow was the best pleasure I had ever known. I loved playing with her and being with her; it just didn't matter anymore if I was fat. It's sad how being overweight changes your life and can rob you of interests and activities.

One day I wore what I thought was a very chic two-piece oversized purple shirt and leggings. I arrived at work—late as usual. Everyone was already around the conference-room table. As I made my way to a seat, one of my male co-workers turned to comment and actually said, "Look, here comes Barney!" All of them, even my boss, burst out laughing. I wanted to crawl under the nearest rock. Instead, I joined in on the fun at my own expense.

As the years went by, I had all but given up hope that I would ever be thin again. I thought I had better accept the fact that I would look like a "matronly housewife" for the rest of my life. Feeling the need to spice up my outlook on life as well as my marriage, I went to Glamour Shots to have my picture taken for my husband. I really looked forward to the photo session and to giving him a picture of myself. I remember thinking that even though I was fat, I was still pretty. After all, my husband often told me that I was "the prettiest fat lady" he knew. (That proves that he loved me, right?) I felt attractive as I sat through the makeup application, the hair-teasing session, and then the photo shoot. This was exactly the kind of boost I needed. I thought how easy Cindy Crawford's job must be. It was so much fun to ham it up for the camera. I couldn't wait to see the elegant me, the old me. I left the photo studio with a renewed sense of self. I was in a great mood and couldn't wait to give my husband his gift. I was imagining that we would be so happy he wouldn't even remember that I had gained one hundred–plus pounds since becoming his bride.

A few days later, I hurriedly drove to the studio to pick up my portfolio. But when I saw the photos, anticipation quickly turned to disbelief. Who was this woman looking back at me from this glossy five-by-seven? They must have made a mistake and given me someone else's pictures—my mother's, perhaps. The reality of what I really looked like was one million light-years away from the mental image I had of myself. I knew I had put on a few pounds, but *this?* It couldn't be. I paid the $250 for my reality check and left the mall with the photos in my purse—along with a gourmet cookie in my tummy and a diet soda in my hand.

I never showed my husband the pictures. Despite the photographer's best efforts, I didn't look like I thought I should—I looked like a heavy middle-aged woman, not a sexy cover girl. This wasn't me; it couldn't be. I wasn't that far gone, was I? *I weighed over 235 pounds in this photo—at age twenty-nine!*

Stop and think about yourself for a moment. Do any of these stories sound familiar to you? How do you see your body right now, today? How do you picture yourself? Is the picture of yourself realistic? Do you have a horror photo like I did, one that shocked the heck out of you when you realized it was *you?* Are you living like I did,

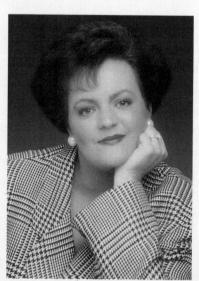

convinced that you are trying your best to lose weight while eating the hamburger and fries? You *have* to eat, right?

Shortly after my modeling career went into its nosedive I started thinking, "I'm pretty, and my body

I think I weighed 235-plus pounds in this photo, at 29!

doesn't look *that* bad." For immediate reaffirmation I'd look around and find someone heavier than I was. It's difficult for me to believe (and admit) that I used to have my young daughter compare me to other overweight ladies. I'd ask her if she thought Mommy was slimmer than *that* lady. We had this nonverbal communication thing going: I would sort of nod in a woman's direction and Taylor would look the woman up and down, then give me her nod. I began getting the "no" nod more than the "yes." I thought I should get the kid's eyes checked; her vision must have been getting bad. At over 235 pounds I wanted to feel "skinny" by some standard, even if my subject for comparison was a woman who weighed over 300 pounds. This made me feel better at the time, but it must have been a confusing self-confidence lesson for my little girl. Don't let your comparison be on the outside; rather, look inside, to discover what you are capable of doing, becoming, and achieving!

Well, a few years later and another twenty-five pounds heavier (which is only about six pounds per year) I was shoe shopping with Taylor when out of the blue a salesperson asked me, "When are you due?" Rather than be a wallflower, I demanded to speak with her manager, and I inquired about training classes in sensitivity for his employees and suggested that this person be sent to one. How dare this woman ask me such a rude question? I was not eight months pregnant! I was full figured, large, plus sized, if you will, but *not* pregnant. I demanded 25 percent off on my shoes. I always seemed to make my problem the fault of someone else.

A couple of weeks later I was relieved to find out that yes, I was in fact expecting. I immediately began telling anyone who would listen, "I'm pregnant!" The translation for this, of course, was "I'm not really fat—I'm pregnant!" I believed that pregnancy would somehow excuse my obesity, or that people would think my fat was all the baby—even though I was only eight weeks along. Maybe that sweet, well-meaning saleslady had been psychic and knew something I didn't. So I went back to doing what I did best: eating for two.

The pregnancy went well. I didn't gain too much weight this time—*only* forty pounds or so. I remember my husband saying to me that if I ended up weighing more than he did he would leave me. It was a joke, of course—I didn't take him seriously. (I think that I had already surpassed his weight anyway.) Why should I take him seriously? We had been married six years now, and our marriage was stable. We had one child and one on the way.

Our lives continued to move along as they had in the past; we had obviously even managed to have sex once in the previous few months. By this point in our marriage my husband was hardly ever around. That was fine with me, as Taylor and I had so much fun together. He didn't know what he was missing! Besides, I had all I needed: a loving child who approved of me and another on the way whom I needed to feed to ensure his growth.

One winter day during the pregnancy, my husband insisted on going deer hunting for what must have been the fifteenth time that month. I put my foot down that Friday night (or Saturday morning, as it was three o'clock in the morning when he made it home) and said, "No, tomorrow you are going to see Taylor sit on Santa's lap with me whether you like it or not. I promised her you'd be there." He refused and called me a few choice names before falling asleep on the couch.

I was upset and felt particularly feisty that night. After finishing my midnight snack, I got out the red food coloring and put some on a cotton ball. I proceeded to paint his nose red—it was brighter than Rudolph's on a cloudy night. I kept thinking that in the morning he would see it in the mirror and know I meant business, then go back to bed and later accompany his daughter to see Santa. I went to bed, only to awaken and find him gone. There was no note telling me where he'd gone. I went about my day. It was a bitterly cold morning, and an hour or so later in comes the deer hunter, panic stricken and actually frightened. He was exclaiming that he was frostbitten, that his nose had gotten frozen while he sat up in his tree stand. He said he had gone back to his truck to warm up when he noticed his very red nose. Then he raced home so that I could take him to the emergency room. His nose was *really* red—he feared he might lose it. I was laughing so hard I fell on the floor. He stood there gazing blankly, like one of his beloved deer with its eyes caught in the headlights of an oncoming car. I held up my fingers, which were also stained red. Slowly it dawned on him that I was the Mother Winter who had caused his "frostbite." It is sad to say that this was one of the few times we laughed together. He never did make it to see Santa. It remains one of our better moments together. I do enjoy a good practical joke.

Clark Leonard came into the world in August, via a scheduled C-section, thank goodness, for at 280-plus pounds I thought labor might have killed me. My best friend, Dana, drove me to the hospital, my parents bringing Taylor along later. The new father made it in time, and stayed around long enough to take a picture or two. He had to leave soon after I was taken to my room, as he had an important dinner meeting at a nice restaurant in town. He was a carpenter, and he had only union meetings to attend. My father couldn't understand what meeting he would have that was more important than getting to know his new baby. I didn't mind because I wanted to get acquainted with my new son.

He was my little "frog baby"; I tease that he resembled a frog when he was born. Taylor came into this world so gorgeous that nurses from other units actually stopped by to see "the precious baby girl." But Clark was all boy—he didn't want to be mistaken for a girl even for a second. He was so long and skinny that his uncle nicknamed him Spindles and made jockey jokes. Again I had gained twice as much weight as is medically recommended in a pregnancy, convinced that it was all baby. My six-pound baby was not nearly big enough to account for the weight I'd gained. He was adorable, he was a life to be loved, and I had now another life to focus on without having to think of my own. With two children, my habits were less important, and I could be a child too—with fewer responsibilities and a lot of fun. Changing diapers and feeding were even fun. Taking the focus off me was a relief—again.

By this point in my marriage I didn't know which I disliked more: the way being with my husband made me feel or the way I felt about myself. He did manage to squeeze in enough time to bring us home from the hospital. He pulled up to the curb in his huge pickup truck, and I had to strain to climb into it. He must have forgotten I had just had a C-section. In any case, we were on our way home.

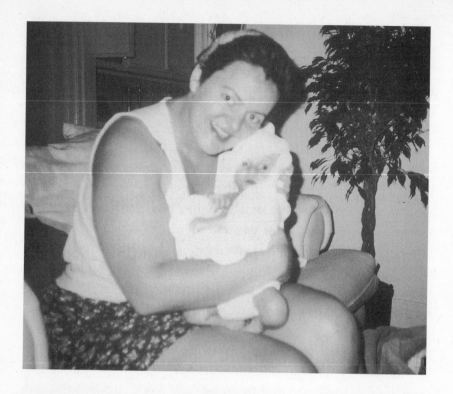

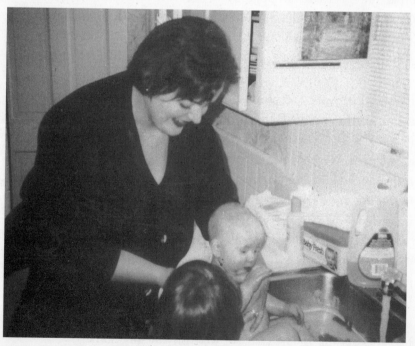

Once home, I found a friend of his lying on the couch in our living room with his new girlfriend. My husband then suggested I make a snack for everyone. I threw a bottle of catsup across the room, packed up the diaper bag, and, against doctor's orders, drove myself to my friend Dana's. Perhaps this was due to a dose of postpartum depression, or maybe just to an insensitive husband. Either way, I was out of there.

The girls and their husbands and all of their kids were at Dana's for dinner. They were much better company and much better caregivers for me and the baby than I had encountered at home. They all marveled at how cute the "frog baby" was. I have the sweetest friends. They told me little white lies to make me feel happy. They were enraged by my husband's lack of sensitivity. All voiced the opinion that I should divorce him. This wasn't the first time I had heard that, but I was in no shape mentally or financially to do it. I tuned them out because I didn't want to listen, no matter how right they were. What did they know? They had perfect lives and husbands who not only loved them but were actually helpful with raising the children, were good providers, and didn't spend more time out with friends than at work. I didn't like my life, but I sure didn't want to make it worse. I believed I wasn't worth any better than I had, and that since I was fat no one else would ever want me.

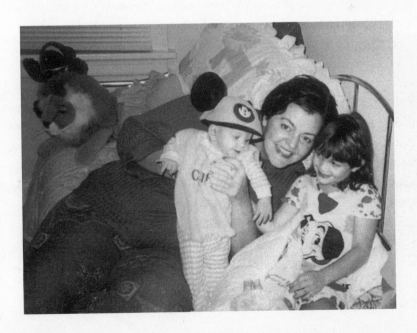

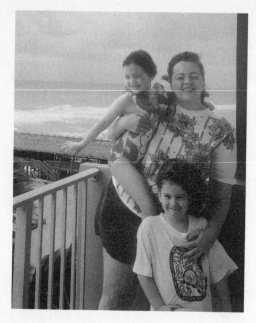

Things continued on in much the same manner for the next few months. My husband was laid off again. He decided this would be the ideal time to remodel our house. With no money, a new baby, and a terrible marriage, he began to rip our house apart. Walls were torn out and "the stairway to nowhere" was built. Weeks went by with very little progress, but there were lots of messes for me to clean up each night when I returned home from work. When I got home it was time for him to leave. He would go to the lumber store and then out for a beer. I found myself alone with the kids much of the time, but I didn't have time to miss him. I had diapers to change, drywall dust to tend to, lots of laundry and cleaning to do—not to mention ice cream to eat and the movie of the week to watch.

I never did weigh myself after having Clark. I weighed 260 pounds prior to my pregnancy and estimate that I topped the scales at 290 just before delivering. Despite the fact that I lost some "baby weight," I know that I gained some fat in the months following the delivery. I just didn't care any longer. My kids didn't care that Mommy was very heavy. They loved me just the way I was. They weren't old enough to know any better. I used to make up bedtime stories to tell the kids about their dad, portraying him as a little-boy cowboy. I did it to give the kids memories that included their dad, to make him bigger than life to them. I really thought that made me a good wife.

My husband and I fought about his absence, yet whenever he *was* around it was so unpleasant, so *why* did I want him home in the first place? Besides, when he was around, I didn't feel like I could curl up on the couch with a half gallon of ice cream for fear that he would make fun of me. I enjoyed it most when I was alone: me, my sitcoms, and my ice cream. I was fine—or so I thought.

The few times I'd see myself in a photo, I couldn't believe or accept that it was me. I didn't look like that, did I? In truth, at this point I would have been thrilled to look as svelte as I had in the Glamour Shots pictures. Although I adamantly refused to allow anyone to take my picture, I accepted a friend's gracious offer to take pictures at my son's first birthday

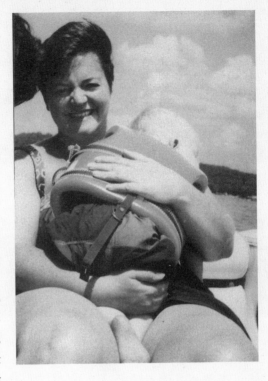

party. It was very sweet of her. The outfit I wore that day was so cute. I had bought a shorts romper from a catalog and had spent days sewing on sequins and pearls. I made it look so pretty and I knew it would look precious. I served a delicious menu with a fabulous cake, and all my friends and family were there. My spouse was even there. We were the perfect family.

I thought everyone must be thinking how happy we were: two kids, a nice house, a new job. The "boys" went off for about an hour, leaving my dad to play host and work the grill. Thank God for my dad, who was always there playing the role of co-host with me. The men returned and rejoined the party. My husband gave Clark a fire truck he'd bought while they were gone. "How sweet," I thought, "he left to go get his son a gift. He might not be the best host, but he loves the kids." It wasn't until months later that I found out the little red fire truck was from his mistress.

A few days after the party my friend gave me prints of the pictures she had taken. "The backstabber—the traitor," I thought. Her pic-

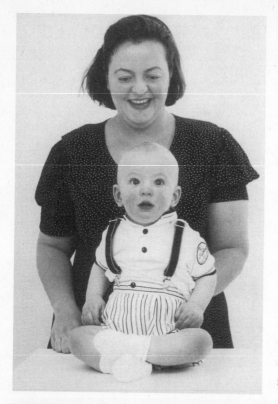

tures revealed the truth: She was no friend. Her pictures made me look absolutely huge. The woman in those pictures couldn't be me! I had been the picture-perfect hostess that day, I'd had the cutest outfit, and the party had been a great success. Who was this obese woman in these pictures wearing my outfit, cutting my son's cake? I was depressed, so I did what I normally did under the circumstances: I reached for something to eat.

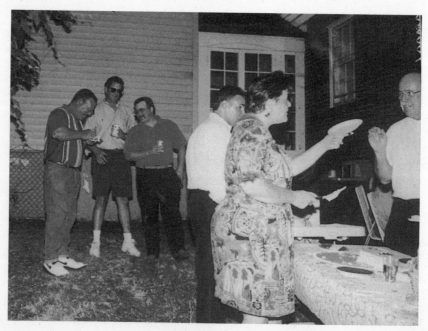

The realization slapped me in the face: My gosh, it's *me*. I was ashamed to think that the thin, young cheerleader and stewardess I used to be had become a matronly, very heavy woman. I was barely thirty years old. So I ate the rest of the birthday cake and pledged to start on a diet—tomorrow.

Life-Changing Events

My "tomorrow" was a long time dawning. It wasn't until I took a good, long look at myself that I realized and accepted the fact that I had become the lady with the large rear end and ill-fitting pants. Makeup wouldn't cover up, and new outfits couldn't hide, my obesity. Looking back, it's easy to see that I hated the way I looked. I have very few pictures of myself holding either of my two precious children. As a matter of fact, very few pictures of me exist at all from my fat years. I was hiding, hiding behind my weight and my unhappiness, for many years.

You already know of the demise of my marriage and how that facilitated my decision to change. While that certainly was a big motivation to change my ways, a few other events also contributed to my wanting finally to lose the weight. Some reasons were more subtle than others, and this one was downright scary.

One afternoon I was at my parents' after the letter about my husband came, seeking their advice as to how I should pick up the pieces of my shattered life. My father was indulging me with one of his wonderful neck massages. He abruptly stopped, announcing that he felt a lump at the base of my neck. Not that he and I are two hypochondriacs, but cancer was our immediate diagnosis. While he planned the funeral, I called my doctor for an appointment. The days in between the fateful discovery and my appointment were terrible. I was filled with fear, anxiety, and regret. I thought of all of the things I wanted to do in life and realized that I had done so few of them. I arrived at the doctor's office a few days later and waited nervously in the exam room picturing the piano-box casket with me stuffed inside, and I worried for my children. Who would raise them? Would they remember me when they were older? Would this other woman raise my little girl, who would then think this woman was her mother? "Clark is so little, he won't even remember me," I thought. As I lay there on the table draped in a paper gown, I was scared. I didn't think of myself as a very strong person; I wouldn't be able to handle this like some of the people you read about, women who battle cancer with such strength and character, overcoming their disease and becoming role models for others in the fight. I was shallow and self-absorbed. I felt as though I had only my loyal friends from high school, my babies, and my father to help me. No one else even wanted to be around me, not even my husband. All those times I spent alone hadn't prepared me for the desperate loneliness I now felt.

The doctor came into the room. He proceeded to ask me the usual symptom discovery questions. How long had I had the lump? Had I been doing anything different? Did I have any pain? He examined me and spent a great deal of time kneading the lump in my neck. It didn't hurt when he touched it—that must be a good sign, I thought. He instructed me to get dressed and to meet him in his office. "Uh-oh," I thought, "so much for good news."

As I sat in his office looking in awe at the physician's many diplomas and certificates, I became even more frightened. He obviously knew his stuff, and he must have known right away that I had cancer and must be about to proclaim my death sentence. He finally walked in and slowly made his way to his chair. He took a deep breath and told me, "This is not what you are going to want to hear, Julia. The lump is a . . . fat deposit." He went on to add that I needed to lose weight. He recommended that I start modifying my eating habits and start exercising.

Now I actually *wanted* to die. Cancer would have sounded better to me at that moment. I couldn't even get dying right. What a mess— a joke. I remember thinking, "Everyone makes fun of me and everyone has been laughing at me behind my back for years." More negative thoughts began to race through my head. Then it dawned on me that I had abused myself more than anyone else had. Here I was, thinking I had cancer, only to find out the "illness" was of my own making. I started to think that the problems in my life might actually be of my own making, a concept I just couldn't handle. If the diagnosis had been cancer, much of the treatment and recovery would have been out of my control. I would have been somewhat helpless over my destiny. I wondered if a person who had been told that she had cancer would trade places with me at this moment, or I with her. How would she feel when told that her disease could be reversed—if only she changed her eating habits, exercised, drank plenty of water? These were deep questions for me, and the answers were even more disturbing. I needed a diversion.

Not to worry. On the way home I swung by my favorite pastry shop: It was amazing how my thoughts cleared after a napoleon or two.

Even then I didn't change. I wanted to, and I even thought I was changing. I was eating less—only sweets, rather than a meal with sweets. I knew how unhappy my life was as I spiraled out of control. It was pretty pathetic.

To add more insult to my injured sense of self, one night, after getting the kids to bed and having done all of my housework, I went for a drive. I had to get out of there, but I really had no destination in mind. I just drove. I couldn't stand to be in the same house with my husband. I went to my favorite park, where there are beautiful old Victorian mansions, huge homes filled with happy families— reminders of the 1901 World's Fair. It is a tranquil place. I lived there when I was single, when I thought I had the world by the tail. I began thinking, "What happened to me to make me end up this way? I used to have so much fun and I really enjoyed life. I had so much energy I used to ride my bike all over the park just for fun." I longed for my old way of life, and I longed for the old me.

On the way home I stopped at a gas station for a candy bar; I had a thing for Mounds bars. I got out of my car, giving my shirt the obligatory tug, thus ensuring that my rear end was well hidden from view so that no one could see I was overweight. This is when I encountered a man I will never forget. I paid for the candy bar at the little window, the one that the cashier slides open, keeping you and the thieves outside. As I turned to walk to the car I noticed this man sitting by the building. He had a brown bag in his dirty, city-stained hands. He looked up at me and smiled. I felt guilty buying candy when the poor man probably didn't even have dinner, or maybe even a place to sleep. I sheepishly looked away. He wasn't about to let me off that easy. As I made my way to the car, giving another tug at my sweatshirt, he shouted to me, "Girl, you got too much food in you! That's right, too much food in you!" The people filling their cars with gasoline immediately burst into laughter. The man continued his heckling: "Too much food!" This man, with nothing to his name, was interfering in my business! How dare he? I got in my car and, I am ashamed to admit, raised a finger, *the* finger, as I drove away. To think that I had actually felt sorry for him—that is, until he opened his mouth. "You old fool, you bum," I thought. I soothed the sting of my humiliation with the delicious coconut filling. As soon as I had driven far enough away that I was sure no one who had heard him would be able to see me, I cried. I cried and thought of what he had said. I thought about my life, and I cried for what seemed like hours.

This may be when I hit bottom. My life had to change because I felt it couldn't get any worse. Even if it could, I knew I couldn't feel any worse about myself. The pain was enough for me to realize that I didn't want to feel this way anymore.

I think about that man often. He was right. He didn't lie, he didn't slander me, he didn't say it to hurt my feelings. He was merely calling it as he saw it. This man was just observant of the world around him, and he has to be to protect himself. I imagine his survival depends on his skill of observation. If it is going to rain, he needs to seek shelter. If someone dangerous looking is approaching him, he needs to hide. He was right. He didn't deserve my gesture. He pointed out what was wrong with me, and he was right. I had too much food in me, plain and simple. He didn't say I was an ax murderer, a thief, or a child abuser. He merely said I had too much food in me. He didn't know I had a marriage that wasn't working, or problems with acceptance. All he could tell was what he could see with his own eyes. I was self-destructing by stuffing myself way beyond capacity. I had too much food in me. I realized then that my problems were caused by my own decisions and that it was time to take responsibility for myself. Maybe somebody had sent this man to wake me up, because he did.

Here is a visual image to illustrate the too-much-food theory. It is a pretty simple concept if you think about it. You pour water into a glass; it fills up. If you keep pouring and don't stop when it is full, it will overflow. The human body, unfortunately, isn't as efficient at getting rid of extra food as the glass is at letting out excess water. Our bodies store it up—in big globs tucked under our skin. You've seen it: It's orange-peel-like in appearance. The old master painters had a gift for making obese women look like beautiful cherubs. That is great for artwork, but in a bathing suit, in today's society, it just doesn't look healthy.

You now know of the many events (you may be feeling like you know too many!) in my life that led up to my finally changing and taking control over my life and my body. I realize this isn't yet enough information for you to be able to do the same things I did. You will get all the details about how I overcame my obstacles and the plan that I followed, but first you need to tap into the "diet within you" and figure out all of the reasons why you want to change. Without doing this and first figuring out your "whys," the forces driving you, all the "hows" in the world won't help you. To get you to the same point I reached, the point when the "why" becomes the driving force behind your future success, you will need to spend time doing some discovery. You must look inside for your motivation and drive to succeed before you embark on any change. It has been said that your "why" for doing something is almost everything, making your "how" as plain as your hand in front of your face. Let's get started with that, shall we?

PART II

Awareness

You Are *Not* Your Body

Are you fat? Answer the question for yourself, and keep the answer in the back of your mind. We will return to your answer in a minute. Now, think back for a moment and imagine how I must have felt when the homeless man was shouting out his observation about my body. How would you feel if that happened to you? Or how have you felt when something similar happened to you? What would you do? Have there been times in your life when someone made a cruel remark or a cutting observation? How did you react?

Now, without emotion, look at your body. Take a long look. Do you see that it has "too much food" in it? Grab a pencil.

Let's assume you said yes to my questions; after all, you are reading a "diet" book. Please write down your answers to the following questions:

How long has your body been overweight? _____

How many diets have you tried in the past five years? _____

Why didn't they work? _____

_____

_____

If they did work, why weren't the results permanent? _____

_____

_____

Why are you here today, reading this book? _____

_____

_____

Think about your answers to these questions and be as honest with yourself as you can. We don't always know the answers, but thinking about these things helps you become more aware of your "whys" so that your "hows" will have a strong foundation of determination. The "why" will be the driving force in your success.

Awareness is essential to your success because it makes rationalization impossible. Rationalization is a tool we have all used from time to time to make ourselves feel better about situations. We can rationalize our weight by telling ourselves that we really have tried to diet and it just didn't work, therefore enabling ourselves to eat half the cheesecake without feeling guilty. You are not alone. We have all been there. We also rationalize the appearance of our body, telling ourselves that we aren't *that* fat. We have all looked in the mirror, strategically moving around until we get just the right angle so we can strike the perfect pose and tell ourselves, "Not bad." But now it's time to put the rationalization aside. It's time for you to cancel your membership in the society for fat acceptance. This is not to say that you shouldn't like yourself regardless of your weight; to the contrary, that is exactly what you should do. The difference is that you must accept *you*, but reject your fat.

I got a very nasty E-mail one day from a woman who was upset with my message. She thought it was terrible that I was telling people to diet and that I should tell them to like themselves despite their weight. I tried to explain that I agree wholeheartedly with her. Yes, we should like ourselves and be happy with the person we are. But our body is not who we are, but what we have. We need our bodies in order to continue living.

Therefore, it is our responsibility to take action to live a healthy life. Think of this analogy: You are given an automobile when you're born to get you around, to go everywhere you want to go. When this auto breaks down, your only focus becomes fixing it, otherwise you won't be able to go anywhere anymore. One breakdown after another finally results in a vehicle that is no longer drivable. That's it. You don't get another one. You're done running errands, visiting relatives, taking kids to the park, traveling the country, going on vacation. Eventually some kind of a breakdown is bound to happen, but if you take care of your vehicle, you have the chance to experience all those things that are a joy not only for you, but also for others because of your ability to express who you are! Don't you want to take care of what you have been given so you can live well and enjoy your life?

Take care of and improve that which is in your ability to control. Getting healthier only enhances your life; it is in no way a bad thing. Accept the best that life has to offer you and *you* will have more to offer.

On my Web site there is a survey where people are asked to list ten adjectives they would use to describe themselves. Please take a moment to do this exercise.

TEN ADJECTIVES

1. _____   2. _____

3. _____   4. _____

5. _____   6. _____

7. _____   8. _____

9. _____   10. _____

When I first read the answers on my Web site, I was very surprised by the words people used. It became evident to me that, regardless of our weight, much of our self-worth and personal esteem is based on the appearance of our bodies. (And I thought I was the only one!) It may or may not surprise you to know that very often when reading the ten adjectives sent in by women wanting to lose anywhere from ten pounds to one hundred or more, I see words like *fat, ugly, gross, obese,* or *chunky*. These are negative, self-deprecating words. While these words may describe what women see in their physical beings, what we are looking for here are words that describe who you are, and what traits make you unique, special, and wonderful.

A woman once sent me the following answers: "fat, ugly, obese, globby, chunky, talented, and sad." She mentioned in her letter that she was a young actress in New York City and that it was becoming unbearable for her to appear in the play in which she was currently cast. Her role was that of a fat woman, and her lines called for her co-star to proclaim that "her heart was as big as Texas" as she was bending over with her rear end facing the audience. I could envision the scene, the entire audience breaking into laughter and her heart sinking a bit deeper with each laugh. My heart went out to her. I responded and told her that I could not accept most of her adjectives, that they were too negative and dwelled on her physical being. I told her that she must think hard and do them over. Five days went by before I again heard from her, this time with a much different response. She said that each time she sat down to write different adjectives, she cried.

Finally, after many hours of soul-searching, she came up with the following list: "magical, spiritual, emotional, sensitive, kind, talented, dreamer, gifted, blessed, and thankful." She said that now it was just a matter of time until her body caught up with who she was on the inside. She vowed to start taking better care of her body and to quit indulging in self-pity. I couldn't have said it any better myself. I am confident that this young woman will get fit and will reach all of her goals. (If she is reading this: I want to be your guest when you are nominated for your first Tony or Oscar!)

What was your answer when I asked, Are you fat? Remember, I did not ask if *your body* was fat; I asked if *you* were. I believe there is a difference. Review your list of adjectives. If there are any negative words on your list, go back, cross them out, and think of some that describe you better.

To further illustrate the concept that we are *not* our bodies, I have another image for you. Picture in your mind's eye the handsome, strong, and striking character Superman as portrayed by Christopher Reeve. His physical characteristics led him to be cast as the ideal man. Today, Reeve has proved himself to be a real-life superhero through his strength of character, his determination, his drive—his own special magic. That magic makes him who he is. It's magic that is in no way dependent on his body or how it looks or functions. I would like to think that he would agree with my statement "We are *not* our body."

Do not lose sight of what we humans are capable of despite the condition or appearance of our physical being, for it is only one small facet of what we are made of. What is inside each of us is far more meaningful than our appearance. We need to rid our bodies of excess fat so that we can live long and healthy lives, not so that we can be better people. Therefore we must not allow our bodies to be anything less than as healthy as we can make them. For those of us who have allowed our body to become obese, that means ridding ourselves of excess fat or of "too much food." We need our body in order to live, so we must take care of it and not give in to being overweight. Life will present many health conditions that are out of our control, so it only makes sense to do what we can to ensure the best function of our body that is within our control.

The problem with accepting our fat as part of us and who we are is that we rationalize away the need to address it and to change. One of the biggest rationales we use for our weight problem is to tell ourselves that we are eating normally and can't figure out why we're overweight. That makes us think that it is not our fault, that we are genetically predisposed to obesity, or that there is nothing we can do about our weight. It is an increasing trend in society to accept obesity as a fact of life, as an irreversible condition. I reject that concept and urge you to as well.

The rapidly rising obesity rates worldwide correlate with the increasing popularity of fast-food establishments, pizza chains, high-sugar soft drinks, all-you-can-eat buffets, and twenty-four-hour doughnut shops, to name a few. Simple awareness of what these "normal" eating habits do to your body will make you think twice before setting foot in (or driving through) places that promote them. I am amazed when someone tells me that dieting just doesn't work for her, yet she is frequenting fast-food restaurants, eating unhealthy foods, and drinking soft drinks. In one of my Take It Off with Julia on-line chats, a woman complained that she was on a plateau and was getting frustrated. I asked her if she had been following her plan 100 percent. Her answer was no. I explained that you cannot change the math. One plus one will always equal two, and the Julia Theorem, $HF+W+E$ will always equal WL (Healthy Food + Water + Exercise = Weight Loss), will never fail.

Since the creation of the first "diet," mankind has associated giving up unhealthy foods with denial. The reality of the situation is that when you eat unhealthy foods and indulge in junk, *then* you are denying yourself. You are denying your body and your life optimal health and the long-lasting benefits of such a life. Passing up a hot doughnut is *not* denying yourself; it is placing yourself one step farther on the path of Self-Improvement through Self-Motivation. It is placing yourself first. If you think about it from this point of view, how could you rationally opt to eat some of the junk offered to us today?

Do you have too much of the wrong food in you? Have you lost control over the appearance of your body? Have you caught a glimpse of yourself naked lately? Don't let this sight upset you too much; *very few* people, even thin ones, possess the "perfect body" without clothes on (sometimes supermodels or Playmates do, and they often have the benefit of airbrushing). Even if you have avoided that sight, *you* know how you look. You may be able to hide from it all day, but *you* know. It is time to take an honest inventory and give yourself a state-of-the-union speech. It is important to define where you are today and what you want to improve upon. Lay out a plan of action first. Then you can take action. Along with a plan to follow, you should also create a realistic mental picture of what your body could look like. This mental image is an important tool as you venture along your self-improvement journey. This image will have a positive, self-empowering, snowball effect on your life. Soon, the reflection staring back from the mirror will be closer to the one you are visualizing today. Before you know it, you will *love* looking in mirrors and will feel proud of the slimmer, healthier, and happier person smiling back at you! Rather than hiding behind rationalizations and loathing yourself for it, you are going to start *now* treating your body and mind with respect. The better you treat yourself, the more dignity and respect you demand for yourself, the more you focus on the quality of life, the better you will naturally treat your body. By adopting this mind-set and creating positive change in your life today, you will feel so much better about yourself. "Change will do you good." You will believe in your ability to succeed with each small step you make toward your goal.

Each step you take in the direction of bettering your health is an accomplishment. Think about how great you feel when you complete a task at hand, or a chore you have been dreading. This is no different!

Tackle your self-improvement project as you would a long-overdue home-repair project. They are very similar. We dread doing it, but once it's done it is great to sit back and admire our work. When I was overweight, it was not only my body that suffered from a lack of attention. My home was a mess, and many other things in life were falling through the cracks and not getting done. There was the needlepoint pillow that I bought, started, and put back into its plastic bag to get to "another day." I would buy a gallon of paint to use in one of the kids' rooms, but by the time I got around to actually using it I had to take it back to have the can reshaken. Even worse, my taste had changed and I no longer liked the color. I spent so much time stressing out over what I needed to get done that little time was left to actually get anything done. Once you make it your policy to start your tasks and complete them, you will feel relieved and gratified.

Each day you take actions that get you closer to your goal is an accomplishment. Be proud of what you have succeeded in, and relish it. Reward yourself for it. Stop beating yourself up over something that happened in the past. Be proud about what you do that *is* right! This can make a big difference in your life. Later I explain how to use a reward system that will reinforce your actions. We set up positive reward systems for our children; when they get an A on their report card, we reward them. When they do their chores, they get an allowance. When they fall short of their objectives, we don't punish them, only encourage them so they can earn their reward.

That carrot-and-stick system doesn't have to be just for kids. You too can be guided by the carrot, and moved a bit by the stick. Pretty soon it becomes second nature, to the point that the mere completion of your goals becomes the reward itself. Many experts say that you need to associate pain with what you are trying to change. That is tough to do when it comes to food and eating. We have to eat to live, so training our mind to associate pain with eating in general just isn't logical. But that doesn't mean you can't associate pain with unhealthy foods. And on the positive side, you can associate pleasure (happiness) with healthy foods.

As you make progress on your self-improvement journey and establish a positive rewards system not only in regard to what you eat but in all areas of your life, then success will be imminent. Your instincts will move you toward that which "feels" good. It just takes time and conditioning. Healthy living will feel better than the way you currently are living. The rewards will reinforce that feeling, and the day will come when you will realize that the true reward is found in simply living your new lifestyle. You will become conditioned to love life and have a passion for it. One of the greatest rewards of this new lifestyle is being able to do and be those things that you feel you have missed out on.

Today, when I tell people of my weight loss, often they don't believe me. I usually hear, "You? No way! You never weighed two hundred and ninety pounds." (As if anyone would want to lie about having been obese— my age, now *that* I will lie about!) I am glad I have a few pictures to show that I was once obese. People often comment that not only am I thinner, but I look ten years younger as

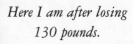

Here I am after losing
130 pounds.

well (maybe that lie will work). My "before" pictures are a good reminder for me and give me an added motivation for staying healthy. I keep my old driver's license in my wallet for a quick reference to my past. I almost don't remember what I felt or looked like at my heaviest weight. Distant are the memories of hiding my face as I shopped at the plus-size stores, or the lonely nights spent in front of the TV eating another half gallon of ice cream. I will never forget the pain of that experience nor the pleasure I have now from living well. As you too will experience, the memories you create with a healthy and fit body will soon overshadow the past painful memories. Being aware of the great differences in those two lifestyles will keep you from ever slipping back again.

Interesting things happen when such changes take place. Life becomes rewarding and full of surprises. I was out for dinner once with my girlfriends and a six-year-old girl loudly told her mother that she thought I was Baby Spice. Me? A woman who not long ago weighed over 275 pounds, who felt miserable, whom people called Barney? I almost screamed "Yes!" right there in the restaurant. (Think *When Harry Met Sally*.) I thought, "Well, I guess there's nothing wrong with being sexy and a mother." Today I look better than I did at age twenty-one, and I'll take that any day of the week! I had convinced myself I was going to be matronly for the rest of my life. This is one case where I am very glad I was wrong.

There are so many wonderful life experiences you miss when you're overweight. Are you missing out on things in life that you would like to be doing, simply because you feel you would look ridiculous or wouldn't fit in? Are you sitting meekly by and watching other people live the life you long for? Why do you think America has become the nation of television junkies that we have? It takes less effort to watch someone do something and be excited about it than actually doing it ourselves. But is that more fun or more rewarding? I don't think so. Do you think Mark McGwire would have had the same feeling watching Sammy Sosa try to break the Roger Maris home-run record if he had not actually experienced doing it himself? Which is more fun and fulfilling: doing something outstanding yourself or watching others do it? Making your *own* great accomplishments or enjoying those of others? Knowing you've overcome the hurdles involved to realize your achievements or watching someone else overcome adversity to achieve the same goals? If you have only watched, make it an inspiration for you to reach your goals.

Don't be a spectator in life—be a doer. If you follow my basic guidelines, you will have the opportunity to do everything on your wish list. Each day, from now on, you will be using your energy to get back into life. It's time to be an active player, not a spectator watching others have fun.

I am trying to inspire you to make changes. Soon you will have the motivation. Then the plan will be yours with which to take action!

Going snow skiing, racing down the slope of a mountain, the wind rushing through your hair, your adrenaline flowing—that is one heck of a lot better than the filling of a pastry. If you don't believe me, try it, and then tell me I was wrong. I promise you, the excitement will amaze you.

Ben Franklin, one of our Founding Fathers, had a great method for problem solving (or at least I heard he was the inventor of this method). He would take a piece of paper and draw a line down the middle. In the left column he would write all of the pros involved in the decision, and in the right column he would write the cons. I want you now to create a chart regarding all the pros and cons of staying overweight and unhealthy versus the pros and cons that you would realize by getting fit and healthy. It seems silly to think that you will be able to name things that would be good about remaining overweight, but there must be something keeping you in your current situation. Take some time to do this exercise and you will be surprised by what you discover.

STAYING OVERWEIGHT

PROS   CONS

1. _____   1. _____

2. _____   2. _____

PROS	CONS
3. _____	3. _____
4. _____	4. _____
5. _____	5. _____
6. _____	6. _____
7. _____	7. _____
8. _____	8. _____
9. _____	9. _____
10. _____	10. _____

GETTING FIT, HEALTHY, AND THIN

PROS	CONS
1. _____	1. _____
2. _____	2. _____
3. _____	3. _____
4. _____	4. _____
5. _____	5. _____
6. _____	6. _____
7. _____	7. _____

PROS	CONS
8. _____	8. _____
9. _____	9. _____
10. _____	10. _____

When you have any decision to make in life, this exercise is a great tool you should use to assist you in making up your mind which way to proceed. As you do the exercise, one column starts to take over and clearly holds the answer as to what path is best to take. For me, the decision was made easier when I looked at the black-and-white facts laid out in front of me. This was the list I wrote out many years ago when I started on my journey:

STAYING OVERWEIGHT

PROS
1. Can hide behind fat
2. Don't have to buy new clothes
3. No exercise
4. No dieting
5. No dating
6. People feel sorry for me
7. People judge me as lazy— won't expect much from me
8. Low expectations of self
9. More "free time" to be lazy
10. _____

CONS
1. Unhealthy
2. Never wear a size 8 again
3. Poor health
4. Poor nutrition
5. Lonely, no dating
6. People think I am cocky
7. People think I am lazy
8. Low expectation of self
9. Less productive
10. Self-doubt

GETTING FIT, HEALTHY, AND THIN

PROS
1. More energy
2. Better body
3. Sexual confidence
4. Longer life
5. Healthier meals, better example for kids
6. Size 8
7. Dating!
8. Great clothes
9. Feel attractive
10. Self-respect

CONS
1. What to do with more energy
2. What to do with longer life
3. Have to buy new wardrobe
4. Dating—arghh!
5. Nothing to blame failures on
6. _____
7. _____
8. _____
9. _____
10. _____

If you can relate to any of the above, take time to really picture yourself—on both sides, so you feel not only the pleasure that will come with the pros, but also the pain that will come with the cons. Remember, this is your list and your life. You can learn from mine, but you must make your own. Don't waste any more time. Maybe that should be one of the pros at the top of your list: more productive and active time, the other side being wasted time, or time spent without energy.

If you can step back from your life and take an unemotional look at the pros and cons of the given situation, the answer as to how best to proceed will be easy to see. Sometimes all we need is a new and fresh perspective on a situation. Doing this exercise will give you just that. Sometimes just looking at the big picture of the facts regarding the situation is helpful. Do not dwell on what was or has been; instead, use this information to facilitate change.

The changes you can bring about in your life will amaze you. I do so many things that just a few short years ago I only dreamed of doing. Silly, fun things like going down the slide at the park with my children, or jumping on a trampoline with them. Remember that I mentioned I had so few pictures of me with my children when they were little? After losing most of the weight, I actually asked someone to take a picture of me with my children. That was a great "pro" of losing weight. I felt pretty and fit, and when I saw the picture I was pleased. I am now in the pictures taken at holidays and events. I participate in the games of football, the softball games, and the ice skating. My life is active now instead of my just sitting back and wishing it were. It is a great feeling knowing that you are creating a picture of life that you can look back on and be happy with. Setting a good example for children is also another pro.

Be proud of yourself that you have realized the right way to live now, before it is too late. Recognize that you are starting today to take the steps necessary to improve your health. Awareness of your actions is the first and most important step. That is all that is required of you now, in order that you may *awaken the diet within you.*

I know that never in a million years would I make one of my best friends sit down in front of the television and force her to eat a gallon of ice cream and follow it with a liter of soda. Yet I did that repeatedly to myself. It was high time I started to think about and treat myself as I would my best friend.

Isn't it time you start treating yourself as though you were your own best friend? Spare yourself further agony. You will see how easy managing what you eat can be. I am living proof that what I did works. I

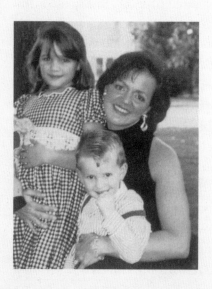

This photo was taken after most of my weight loss, and I was feeling a sense of peace and happiness with my home and family. I was so happy to be with them having my picture taken.

have lost over 130 pounds and have kept most of it off for over six years at this writing. I must be on to something that the "experts" haven't figured out yet.

Many estimates report obesity as a disease, ranking it the second leading cause of *preventable* death in our country. How can something be a disease yet be preventable? If you can prevent something yet you still do it, it is then self-inflicted. Don't overload your body with too much food and you won't be obese. I wish cancer were that easy to cure. As a society we spend billions of dollars a year on weight-loss products and programs, yet we continue to get fatter.

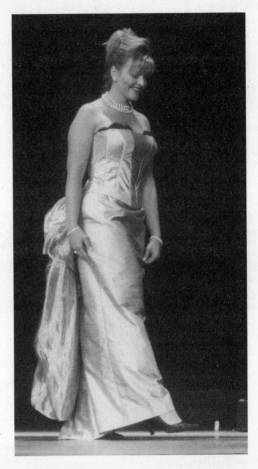

In Las Vegas, evening gown competition, Mrs. United States Pageant 1999.

Decide on a Lifestyle, Not a Diet

The first thing you should understand about weight loss is that focusing on "dieting" is a waste of time and energy. Put your efforts into something really important—your family, your job, a hobby—not a diet. Food no longer needs to be a source of fun. That is a great feeling—and it's the key to successful weight loss. Food has to become less important. You need to focus on yourself and the contributions you make in your own life and to the world around you. You have God-given talents and contributions to make in this world—don't let them go untapped. Live the life, not the diet.

One of the great revelations I became aware of about my lifestyle was that I was eating a lot of unhealthy, fattening foods. I was eating things I thought were healthy, only to find out that they were calorie- or fat-filled. Once I cut out some of this food and replaced it with more healthy choices, the weight started melting off with less effort than I had put forth in numerous previous diets. Best of all, this time I had no crazy diet to follow. If you weigh 250 pounds or more, you are probably eating unhealthy foods—a lot. Cut back on the portions, eliminate some of the fat, and you will be amazed at how easily the weight comes off. Talk about pros!

Many times we mindlessly eat and are not even aware of what we are doing or how quickly those nibbles add up. You know what I mean. You are cleaning up the dishes after dinner and a bite of macaroni is on one child's plate. You begin hearing your mother's voice from your childhood, and you pop that bite in your mouth so you "do not waste food." There may be one piece of pie left in the tin, so rather than taking the time to wrap it up and save it (too much effort for just one piece), you eat it so that you don't have to throw it away. There are two options: Get a maid to do your dishes and let *her* get overweight— or become aware of your actions and stop the mindless eating.

The need for more awareness about your lifestyle can be seen in the results from past dieting efforts. How many times have you said to yourself, "I'll eat whatever I want today and start my diet tomorrow"? You know the result: You binge all day, starve yourself the next, eat moderately on day two, and by day three you can no longer resist having a candy bar or other "forbidden" food. After eating the forbidden food, you think, "Well, I blew my diet now, so I might as well eat anything I want." So you eat everything in sight. Disgusted with yourself, you vow to "go back on your diet tomorrow." But tomorrow never comes. Be aware of what you are doing and its effects on your body. You must believe that you can change and that you can take control over your life and body. Awareness makes this possible— being aware that you *can* make the right decision, being aware that each action *does* make a difference.

I met with one of my readers who happens also to live in St. Louis, a woman I'll call Carol. Her weight was 275 pounds. She E-mailed me and complained that she had tried everything under the "dieting sun" and nothing worked. When an attempt did work, it didn't work permanently, because she was now obese again. She asked me, in a rather disbelieving tone, "What makes you different? What makes your approach any different from anyone else's and wouldn't it just be a waste of my money?"

I went on the offensive and said that I would like to help her change her life—forever. We met for coffee and talked for two hours. I found out many relevant things about what she was doing that enabled her to maintain her 130-plus pounds of extra weight.

For one, she was drinking ten regular sodas a day—ten! That is outrageous, yet at the same time it is all too common. She had absolutely no idea that her soft-drink habit was the biggest culprit in her losing weight-loss battle. One can of soda has an average of 150 calories, and that doesn't take into account supersize portions. Carol was mindlessly sipping away at 1,500 calories a day. To make matters even worse, I pointed out that it takes 20 minutes of cardiovascular exercise to burn off 150 calories. I asked her if she was doing at least 200 minutes a day of exercise. She laughed. She didn't even do 20 minutes. You do the math.

She asked me to help her lose weight and to tell her what to do. She expected me to prescribe a strict diet for her to follow. I now laughed. I asked her, "Haven't you tried those things in the past with little result?" I suggested we try something different this time. I did not ask Carol to change everything about her life and her habits all at once. I asked her to be more aware of what she was doing and the effect it had on her body. I suggested that she work on one thing at a time. Kicking the soda habit would be a great start. She decided to go cold turkey and break her ten-can-a-day habit. It was not easy for her. She made it through one week (and didn't kill anyone, I am pleased to report) without having even one soda. In her second week, she decided to have one at a party she was hosting. She poured it into a glass and sipped on it, then poured half of it away. She said that it felt really empowering to prove to herself that she didn't have to have it. After three weeks, she really wasn't tempted anymore and then when she stepped on the scale for her weigh-in and saw that she had lost seven pounds, she vowed never to drink soft drinks again. Without changing anything else about her lifestyle—only giving up her biggest vice—Carol lost seven pounds in three weeks (that could be twenty-eight pounds in three months). That was just the beginning of her self-improvement journey. That first step led Carol to make other positive changes. She became much more aware of all of her actions and their effects on her body.

Another point for you to become aware of is the concept of time. Today is the very best time to start making positive changes in your life. Right now is when you must start on your self-improvement journey. Strike the "tomorrow is the perfect time to . . ." thinking from your mind. We almost set ourselves up for failure by thinking that we'll start tomorrow—and that we will notice great results soon thereafter.

Recently I gave a copy of my book and some multivitamins and supplements to an acquaintance. I saw him a few days later and asked how it was going. He told me, "Great. I'm going on my diet tomorrow, Julia." He explained that he had "cheated" at breakfast that morning and now "the day was shot," thus making tomorrow the time to restart his diet. The problem for him was that he continually "messed up" today and was always waiting for tomorrow to arrive to try again. I suggested that he just get back on track *now*, rather than waiting. There is not a clock, or a position of the sun, that needs to determine when we start making healthy decisions. Again, I am not talking about a diet, I am referring to a *lifestyle*. Just because he made a poor decision and ate a doughnut does not mean that he needs to put himself in a "diet penalty box" and binge on other unhealthy foods—all in preparation for the new diet day dawning tomorrow. He should have opted to make his next choices healthy ones. When learning to ride a bike, if you fall down, you just get up and try again. You might still be learning to ride if every time you fell down you put the bike away and didn't try again until the next day. This is a journey of self-improvement, one that will be filled with stumbles, challenges, rejoicing, spills, and thrills. Expect them all and prepare to handle them—and start by being aware that they exist.

Deciding that you will start making healthy decisions now is an essential step to living a healthy life. Doesn't this approach seem slightly more logical than *announcing* the start of a diet? "Attention Kmart shoppers, I am on a diet. Yes, that's right, starting this morning in aisle three, I am now on a diet!" That is just silly. It doesn't matter what you ate ten minutes ago, three hours ago, or three years ago, because you can't change it—it is in the past. So forgive yourself, move past it, and get on with changing your life and your body. The only thing that matters is what you eat next or what you don't.

You can't change or control what is in the past; you're able to control only what you decide to do in the present and future. Right now, today, is the first day of the rest of your life. How do you want to live it, and what kind of body do you want to live it in? Your next action does not need to focus on eating something healthy—or on eating at all. It could be to take a walk, ride a bike, or focus on something or someone else that will take the focus off food, even writing down your goals for the week. Any action that you take should be a move in the direction of better health.

Determination

How do you stop the unhealthy cycle in which you find yourself? I know that for me the change was brought about by a collection of humiliating experiences. I don't have all the answers, but I do know this: If today you start caring about yourself more than you do about food; care about your health, realizing that you are in control of what goes into your mouth; begin taking pride in your appearance and living with a meaningful purpose in life, then each day it will get easier to make these right choices about what you eat, and in all that you do. You've got to picture the person inside, the one you know can accomplish great things in life. By calling on the energy deep inside you to break the barriers holding you back from doing anything you want, you will move mountains. You can opt to wait until you have had enough humiliation that it forces you to change, or you can choose to do so now. You can wait until you get a serious health condition, such as diabetes, that scares you into change, or you can decide to change now. You can become a statistic in the increasing number of obesity-related deaths or you can change before that becomes your destiny. If you choose to change, you will. You will improve your health, better your life, and create more joy in it.

Let's begin today. What should you do right now to get started? You've been reading for quite some time and you aren't skinny yet? This book must not work! You're thinking, "Julia doesn't know what the heck she is talking about." You want to get a refund, right? No, you're not thin yet, but guess what? You will be. It will take you time to become educated, to make healthy choices, and to allow the scale to reflect change. But already you have made progress: You have been focusing on *you* and not food while reading this, and that's a great start. I want you to start thinking, and becoming more aware and more educated, about what you need to do—and, most important, taking the actions that will bring you success. Ultimately, all of this is up to you. I can be your coach or inspiration, but you are the only one who is able to stop yourself from eating that next cheeseburger or pastry. You are the one who will be picking yourself up and becoming more active.

Each day remember: Every moment prior to this one is a moment lived—it becomes a memory. But this moment, right now, is one in which you can make the decision to think positive thoughts, choose healthy food, and tap into your innate abilities and talents. After all, "Today *is* the first day of the rest of your life!"

Don't let another day or moment go by without taking one small step toward improving who you are. Just by making one small positive and healthy choice, you can see magnificent changes in just two weeks.

Imagine that there are things you would do, or ways in which your life would be different, if only you were more fit. Write down three of the most important ones:

1. _____

2. _____

3. _____

How does reading this list make you feel? Do you want them so badly you could scream? We all imagine that the grass is greener on the other side of the fence. The grass *is* greener on the other side only because you are too busy watching theirs to care for yours properly. The beauty of this concept when applied to weight loss is that if you do these things right now you will realize your weight-loss dreams much sooner. You don't have to wait until you are thin to go to the park, to go swimming, to take an exercise class—you can do it now. These activities will only help you reach your goal more quickly. The things that you want out of life as a thinner person are easily attained—and actually doing those things *now* helps to make you thinner and healthier. Then the little black dresses and smaller-size jeans will follow.

An eighteen-year-old woman who weighed 330 pounds came to stay with me for a week—sort of a motivation boot camp. I stressed, among other things, that she needed to start living her life now, not wait until the day the scale reached a certain number. I told her, as I am telling you, that she must step out of her comfort zone and start living. Doing those very things would help her to realize her fitness goals. When she returned home, she called me and told me of an upcoming rafting trip that her church group was planning. She really wanted to attend but felt she was too big. I practically forced her to go. She went reluctantly. She called a few days later to tell me how much fun she had and thanked me for encouraging her to go. I asked her if she managed to eat healthfully on the two-day trip and make good choices. She said for the most part she ate healthy foods, but that wasn't the hardest part of the trip for her. You see, she fell out of the raft on the first day. It took three men to pull her back into the raft, and she was mortified. She said, "Julia, after that happened I became so determined not to fall out of that raft again, and I didn't!"

I explained to her that the determination she had mustered for staying in the raft was the very same determination she would need to call upon to help her eat healthier foods and exercise regularly. She was one step ahead of me. She said that the rafting trip had changed her life and that she will go on the trip again, only next time she will be considerably thinner. I am convinced that she will realize her goals. At last report, she had lost forty-five pounds and continues to make steady progress on her path of self-improvement.

Determination is an amazing thing. In the context of weight loss, determination entails visualizing the goal plus taking action toward achieving that goal: Visualization + Action = Results.

The most difficult part of achieving any goal we attempt is getting started. Sometimes, usually when we least expect it, life changes course and forces us into change. When this happens the going may be rough—especially in the beginning. Other times in life, change is brought about by a conscious decision. In either case, once we take command of the new circumstances we can manage to move ahead and create something positive amid the chaos. When I found myself weighing in at 290 pounds, my marriage crumbling, and my self-esteem falling rapidly in a downward spiral, I knew things needed to change. I wasn't sure exactly what I needed to do, but I knew that I wanted my mind, body, and soul to be better off in my future than they were currently. I set about establishing a set of healthy principles to live by.

It is time for you to do the same. If you haven't figured it out by now, my dissatisfaction with my body manifested itself in every aspect of my life. It consumed me. I had become a very negative person. Everything negative in my life was always someone else's fault. I let my self-pity absolve me of all responsibility for my actions. I felt like the world owed me, since my life wasn't turning out at all as I had planned. However, once I realized this and how unhappy it was making me, I decided I wanted more out of my life than I had managed to get so far. I took some serious inventory, I realized a lot of the things about myself that I didn't like, and I decided to change them for the better—forever! That is the great thing about life. We have the ability, at any moment, to make a change, to rewrite our personal screenplay. Change the character you are playing, or give that character a new persona or a new body in which to play it. Make a change that will make you happier.

Happiness comes in many different forms. When we forget that and allow food to become the major source of our happiness, we miss out on so much else that life has to offer. How many times in your life have you jumped on the scale, only to allow your day to be ruined because of your weight? It is almost as though we are purposely upsetting ourselves when we weigh ourselves every day—or numerous times in one day. Just as there are things we do that upset us, there are many things that can make us happy. We need to switch our focus from searching for short-term solutions to looking ahead one day, one week, one year, maybe even a decade or two—and deciding what we want our life to be like. Then we need to decide whether the choices we have made are ones that are going to get us closer to that ideal or continue to push us farther away. The greatest fulfillment in life is to be as healthy, compassionate, and caring as you can be. *That* is true happiness, and it will last you forever. This is the real thing, not a dress rehearsal. This is a huge break from the traditional "dieting advice" you may have thought you were going to get when buying another "diet" book. This is also why this will be the last "diet" book you will ever have to buy, because this approach will allow you to change your mind as well as your body forever. The first thing you must do in order to change is become aware of your positive and negative lifestyle choices.

Take a step back and rationally review your lifestyle. Stop your unhealthy actions, such as eating ice cream and doughnuts, as well as being envious of all the people who are fit. All of our negative actions have repercussions for others. This is a vicious cycle that we're not *aware* of. I know that I was moving through life so fast I didn't take the time to think about what I was doing, or to think about what the consequences of my actions were going to be. I was completely unaware of the person I was at the time, until the person I had become looked in the mirror and said, "This is *not* who you really are or who you want to be!"

What does it mean to be aware of who you are and who you desire to be? Even if you know the kind of fit and healthy person you want to be, don't you need to be aware of who you are now so you know what changes to make for yourself in order to get there? One of the first things to learn about yourself is when your weight actually became an issue. I've read thousand of surveys submitted to my Web site, and it is very interesting to read how many of us, myself included, have similar answers to the question "At what age did you first believe you were overweight?" For most people, it was twenty years earlier. That's a lot of time to be concerned with something yet not actually deal with it. For twenty years you may have been making attempts to solve a weight issue that has only become worse over the years.

Sometimes you travel down a road so far and so long that you are no longer *aware* of why you actually got on the road—and therefore you can't be sure how to get off the road and onto the one that leads to where you really want to go!

Going back to where we actually got on this road that brought us to where we are today can help. Remember, there may be one action that put you on this unhealthy path—one that led to other actions, only to create what seems to be a never-ending road that is going in circles. It's time you find that "on-ramp" to your life again. I want to show you how.

Got that pencil handy? Now I want you to think for a moment.

When did you first get on the path by beginning "not-so-healthy" eating habits? Write your answer below:

_____

What was going on in your life, or what event influenced your actions at the time?

_____

_____

Are you happy heading in the direction you have been going?

_____

Do you want to change the direction of your life?

_____

Now that you have identified and become aware of that time in your life when you may have gotten on this unhealthy path, it is just as important to be aware of all the times you have experienced some pain along the way to today, things that are reminders of the weight you don't want. The three-way mirrors in the clothing stores, or the outfit that no longer fits, the playground you felt you couldn't go on with your kids, or, for me, the comment from across the parking lot. Do these things make you aware that something should be done? I know they did for me, and I'm sure they do for you.

Often, our intentions to lose weight and get fit fail us because eventually the negative feelings we associate with painful events wear off and no longer motivate us to succeed. In fact, oftentimes we can avoid running into these painful events again. You stop looking in the mirror at those clothing stores—you know your size and you don't need to look. You avoid those playgrounds—after all, they can be dangerous. Or how about throwing away those outfits that don't fit— they were out of style anyway. Or, worse yet, you pass up going to re- unions or weddings, saying, "I don't need to show off" or "There is no one there I want to see." When we avoid the situation, we tem- porarily feel better and life can go on again. You must become *aware* of this, because it happens all the time. It happened to me, and I'm sure it has to you. When we allow this cycle to continue, we go on and off diets faster than kids switching rides at the park. So many people have done this so frequently that we even have a name for it: yo-yo dieting.

Being aware that this cycle of events has occurred and keeps oc- curring in your life, from the age you may have believed you had a weight issue up until today, is important so you know what is going on. I am not asking you to remember these painful issues so you can feel bad about them and beat yourself up all over again; carry the memories calmly and objectively and *be aware of them* so you can use them as tools to reshape your life.

Now that you are more aware of where and when the road you are on began, and the painful experiences along the way that led to your unsuccessful weight-loss attempts, you can seek a permanent solu- tion.

It's time that you find your on-ramp, make a *you*-turn and get back on the highway that is *your life*—the life you dream of, not the un- healthy life you may have been living. Right now you are on the ramp. You may have even made the turn. Your intentions in starting this "diet" are sincere. This ramp is uphill, as so many are, so you need the right actions in order to accelerate your movements in the right direction to get on the healthy road.

Stop, Look, and Listen

Remember this phrase: "Stop, Look, and Listen." These three words will help you become more aware of the things you have been letting control you and help you take control of them.

Stop. The easiest thing to remember in times when you may be headed toward doing or eating something that is questionable is to stop. Think to yourself: "Am I going to eat something that may keep me from progressing on the road to fitness?" "Will I be pushing my goals back another day, week, or month?" Start to become aware of your actions before you take them. In other words, when you wake up tomorrow, become aware of what you are pulling out of the kitchen cabinets. Is it healthy or unhealthy? Be aware that if you are in a hurry to get to work or to get the children off to school, it may cause you to cut corners. You may be feeding the kids or yourself fast food or sugar-laden cereal instead of fresh cantaloupe or honeydew and eggs. Become aware of your actions at work. When you take a break and go get a soda in the morning, stop and realize that there is absolutely no nutritional value in it and that it will not contribute to your moving up on your *you*-turn ramp. When it's lunchtime, be aware of what you usually eat and whether it's good for you. *Stop* and change the patterns of your actions. As your day continues, be aware of all the things around you that may be pulling you back or keeping you off the ramp. You will start to notice how many things you actually have control over. *Stop* before taking actions that are not going to keep you on the road to success.

Next, you need to **Look**. As I became heavier over the years, many things in my life were not getting done. I would often leave work

early because I just didn't have the energy to perform. Things everywhere around me were barely getting done. You know what I mean:
The trash can is overflowing to the point where things are all over the
counter, and boxes next to it are becoming little side trash containers.
The dishes build up in the kitchen sink until there are no clean ones
left. I'm talking about looking around your life and taking inventory
of the unfinished jobs and unfinished actions that are present, then
doing the dishes until every last one is clean, taking out the trash—
not just the kitchen garbage but emptying every trash can in the
house. Or how about those tasks at work that have to get done at
some point? Why not try to complete them all today? Get it out of
the way and move on! Look at what you're not getting done and *do it*.
Looking will help you be more aware of the things in your life that
are not getting done, that are cluttering up not only your life, but
your mind as well. Think of five things you must do before your life
is over: skydiving, traveling the world, missionary work, even writing a book.

Now ask yourself, "Are the simple things like cleaning the house,
or completing a project at work, holding me back from doing more
meaningful things in my life?" If you don't learn to complete the
smaller, simple tasks, you won't complete the bigger ones. Look
around your life for things that need to be cleaned, that are acting like
a smudge on the window of your life. Be aware of the tasks you need
to complete and start to see every job as one that needs to be finished
at the very moment it is undertaken. Don't wait for some future date
to plan on doing these things. As you start to do them, you will then
become aware of the time you have to do the things that are more
meaningful—and you'll have the motivation as well.

The next and last step toward increasing awareness is to **Listen**.
Listen to what, you say? You know that voice inside you that may
ramble on about things. I'm talking about your thoughts, those con-
versations we have with ourselves about what to do, when to do
things, whether we like things or not. What am I going to say to my
spouse; how mad I am about that driver who cut me off; that so-and-
so at work who I hope gets fired; or those friends who brought doughnuts—who do they think they are, anyway? Yeah, those thoughts. All

that junk that just doesn't do us any good at any time. Those thoughts influence your actions. They need to change. I remember how much time I had to talk to myself when I was tipping the scale, and how many people and things I "hated." I let my hatred for my body turn me into a very negative person. I don't even like to use that word anymore because it's so harmful. Even things that are bad I don't "hate" but I prefer to avoid, to change, to make different, to do something about, to have a positive influence on, to correct, or to make good.

Do you see yourself as being negative more often than you would prefer? Positive self-talk is the most powerful tool available to you, and it is one that will make a difference in your life. Tell yourself you can accomplish your goals, that you can succeed in all your efforts, that you will lose weight, that you will travel to those far places, that you will do everything on your to-do list before you die—*and you will*. Tell yourself the contrary—I'm not going to mention the thousands of ways you can do so, because you know them—but tell yourself the contrary, and the contrary will happen. Wake up in the morning and make your thoughts positive. Such as, "What a beautiful day. I can't wait to get up and start my day and get things done. What a great opportunity I have today to make my life better, to improve my relationships, to be more productive, to live more happily, to fulfill my dreams. Isn't it great that I have the chance to make today better than yesterday? All of the things that need attention, I can give attention. Today I can smile and say hello to all the people around me, no matter what their mood or how unfriendly, because I don't need to let anyone else influence what I think about myself or what I think about them."

A wise man, Napoleon Hill, once said: "If your mind believes it, then you can achieve it." Listen to your thoughts and make them positive ones, no matter how tough the situation, no matter if frustration comes your way. Change the way you think about what you need to do and who you want to be. After all, the only difference between what may be a bad day and what is a great day is your perception. If you were faced with nothing but difficult challenges today, you can either be mad and unhappy about it or grateful that you had the opportunity to face these challenges in order to grow as a person. Learning how to deal with adversity and becoming aware of how you handle any situation is a strong and powerful educator that will keep you on the positive highway that should be your road for life, one that keeps you moving toward the person who is healthy, fit, happy, and successful.

As you start getting on this ramp to the highway of your life, you will develop good habits. When these habits set in, you will be happier and healthier. Remember, though, that there are many exits and each has its own temptations. You know the ones. Those desserts we have at the holidays, the birthday cakes at the office, or the remainder of your child's PBJ. Think of those times when you are faced with eating some unhealthy foods or skipping your exercise program. Try to remember this image: When you choose an unhealthy action, you have just taken an exit off the highway of health and life!

Don't despair—you can get right back on the highway as long as little time has passed, and I mean little—like only a couple of hours. If you have put yourself at any time in a situation where you have taken one of these exits, be sure you do something healthy within a couple of hours: Take a walk, ride a stationary bike, do any form of exercise. The more quickly you do this, the easier it will be to go right back up that on-ramp to the road of your life. This is the key to long-term success.

Be aware of where you are now. Make the necessary effort to get on the healthy road of your life to where you want to go. And always realize when you have taken an exit off that road, so you can hurry and get back on, because once you get on it, it's much easier to stay than it is to get back again.

We can have awareness, but that isn't enough. We need to also know the basics about health: what foods are good for us, what is healthy, and what we should do to improve our fitness.

From now on, *stop* before consuming anything. *Look* at the item and decide if it is healthy—then *listen* to yourself!

PART III

Awakening the Diet in *You*

Getting Started

I want to begin by pointing out that I don't want to mislead you with the title of this chapter. In every diet program there seem to be changes in lifestyle or habits that are designed only to achieve a specific goal. Once the goal is met, you jump up and down and cheer your success. Oftentimes we celebrate our "diet success" with a big meal, a dessert, and/or a soda—after all, we did it, we finished the diet. We revert back to our previous way of life, the life we know. Certainly you don't want to go through that ever again. Most plans are not designed to be something you can live by for the rest of your life. Just saying it makes me sigh. This is why it is so important to get a few "Julia basics" in place in order to create your own lifelong success.

There are a few areas you should get control of and understand fully. They will build the foundation for your continued success. Getting a firm grasp on this new line of thinking *is* "getting started." I will outline the items you need to grasp as you get started. I will not list an overwhelming number of specific actions you must take every day. That approach would not have worked for me. Think of me as a college professor who teaches a business course that will allow you to have the knowledge to start your own business. Your teacher may also give you examples of her own experiences, good and bad, during her years in business, and what allowed her to succeed, as well as what helped her to get through tough times. Now, can she reach *your* goals for *you*? Of course not. But you can reach them if you take the most pertinent points from the lessons taught to you in life. Those points are necessary for you to get started, to continue, and to make progress one step at a time. When things get tough, remember that it is all a part of making progress.

With that said, I want to discuss a few points that will give you what you need to ensure that you get started and continue on the path of self-improvement. One of my favorite phrases is "We don't plan to fail, we fail to plan." It is important that we have a plan when beginning any project. This project, your Self-Improvement through Self-Motivation journey, may be the most important project you ever start in your life. With that in mind, I want to help you develop the best possible plan that will work for you. In order to develop a plan, you will need to have knowledge and awareness of yourself. Realize that if the same plan worked for everyone, obesity wouldn't be at epidemic proportions. Once your plan is created, you will need to arm yourself with the *inspiration* and *motivation*—the *"why"* to succeed. Then and only then can you put forth the *effort* necessary to *train your mind.* This journey requires *knowledge, training, purpose, motivation*, and *application* in order to keep you progressing on the path of self-improvement. When I lost my 130 pounds, I did not do it thinking that I was creating a method that would help others. I did what worked for me. I became aware of what was bad about what I was doing and what would be better and healthier. Once I learned how horrible some of the things were that I was putting in my body, that awareness made it virtually impossible to continue in the direction I had been heading. The awareness gave momentum to my effort.

Knowledge

There are many so-called experts out there who have created so many books on the subject of health and weight loss that it's hard to believe that every one of us who has read these books or has tried their different weight-loss plans doesn't have a doctorate on the subject. I'm here to tell you that I'm not one of those experts. I'm not going to fill your mind with every fact about calories, digestion, metabolic rates, insulin factors, and so on. If that is what you are seeking, head back to the bookstore.

What worked for me—and for thousands of others—is keeping things simple. Why spend countless hours learning about every fact associated with the body's functions, fat grams, and total calories, when what really matters is creating a high quality of life? I know there are exceptions to the rule, as there always are—perhaps you're diabetic or you have another condition that requires specific nutritional knowledge—but even then you still have to *want* to use the knowledge that can help you.

Your life should not be consumed with thoughts of food and weight loss to the point that you lose the focus of fulfilling your dreams. I remember trying every diet plan and program available. If even one of them worked, I wouldn't have needed any of the others. I became more discouraged with every failed diet, and I was getting more and more angry about other things in my life. My weight was, in many ways, a by-product of these emotions. I was convinced that I, not the diets I put my faith in, was the problem, the failure.

There are things I have learned along the way that are important, and they are worth passing on to you. These are simple yet powerful points that will help you create lasting change. I don't think it will deter your weight loss if you don't fully understand exactly how blood-sugar levels are regulated, or the chemical reaction that takes place when fat is mobilized. In this book you will learn what foods to avoid and what to eat more of, but your education needs to focus more on *you* and what is going to allow you to succeed. Don't get so wrapped up in the details that you're not seeing the big picture: the life you want to be leading.

There are so many different facets of health when it comes to the body's systems, organs, and cells. But there is one organ that is superior to all when it comes to our capabilities and our potential. I am talking about *the mind*, specifically about your beliefs. This is the first, and what I think is the most important, educational fact to grasp in order to succeed in any area of your life. If you take part in any weight-loss program because someone else said it works but you don't believe in your own abilities much less the diet's, then the program won't work! I'm not going to tell you to follow a plan step-by-step and have you blindly believe that it will work for you. I am telling you to believe without doubt that *you* have the ability to reach your goals—all of them. Not because I said so, but because *you* say so. This is the first point you must take home. It is a *must*.

There is one thing that separates someone who is accomplishing their goals from someone who is not: The first person began with a belief that they could succeed. Don't be a victim to any excuse, just start with the belief that you cannot and will not be defeated.

I didn't let doubt get in the way of my quest for a better life. I believed that I could change; then when I decided to do it, it finally happened for me. What good is a plan if you do not believe in your ability to implement it? You must begin your journey with the firm belief that you can succeed, or you will miss the most crucial step in reaching any goal. Never doubt your ability, no matter how ambitious the goal or objective may seem.

If you have tried numerous diet attempts before and failed, or even succeeded, only to gain all the weight back again, this is probably hindering your confidence in yourself and your belief in your ability to succeed. If that is the case, let me erase those doubts from your mind by explaining to you why diets don't work. Once you know this, you will realize that it was *not* you who failed, but the diet that failed you.

Why Diets Don't Work

If you are like I was and have been living with these habits for years, with habits ingrained in your mind, with your actions occurring almost automatically, where you are used to giving little to no thought to what you're eating, drinking, or the limited physical activity you are getting, then certainly these habits are going to be difficult to break. If you are living with habits that are keeping you from getting fit, waking up tomorrow to begin a *whole new lifestyle* comprised of a *completely* different eating plan or diet and new habits that start with exercise each day seems absolutely impossible. Yet this is what virtually every diet ever created expects us to do. It's an overwhelming change! Facing this dramatic overhaul all at once makes it almost impossible to stay with your new regimen for the long term, much less actually get started on your first day. I call this "overwhelm."

If your new program is simply a diet supplement or a product that promises weight loss without changing any of your habits or daily actions, will you just take this product or supplement forever so you can go on eating and avoiding exercise? Of course not. Besides, it can't possibly be healthy to continue eating fast food and drinking heavy-syrup soft drinks only because you are taking a diet supplement that supposedly counteracts the effects of these foods.

Commercial diet centers' eating plans, the ones where you buy their food, *will* provide you with a sound plan for short-term success, yet going from your current eating habits to a strict plan is an enormous leap that is usually too difficult to make. You can't eat prepackaged foods for every meal forever, so it is difficult to adopt a lifelong lifestyle change in such conditions.

You've heard it said that it takes time to lose weight and get fit. Well, let's go back one step farther and realize that *it takes time to get rid of each unhealthy habit you have, and time to implement each needed healthy habit.* Give yourself the time to develop the healthy actions that are a part of a healthy life, not just time to lose weight. The great thing with this is that losing weight is a result of those healthy habits. You *will* lose the weight. That is a given. If you don't ingrain positive actions one at a time into your lifestyle, slowly and steadfastly, you'll be overwhelmed and want to throw in the towel. You will jump on the scale three times a day or numerous times a week and be discouraged that the pounds are not peeling off at the lightning speed you desired. If you keep your focus on establishing healthy habits and let nature take its own course, you will realize the weight loss. In the past, if you have merely dieted to lose weight, this is why a diet or product failed you, or allowed you to succeed only to gain all the weight back. This time you must take the approach of changing your lifestyle for life.

Having this knowledge should give you the confidence that you can in fact succeed. You do not need to be disappointed by empty promises; this promise is real. If you take things one step at a time and avoid jumping full force into a new lifestyle, you can slowly and effectively acquire these new healthy and fit habits.

The plan I have for you is a one-step-at-a-time approach that I will outline in Part IV: "The Road Map to Weight Loss and Fitness." However, in order to start fulfilling this healthy lifestyle, you must look inside and first find a few more answers about yourself.

Purpose

When I look back at my life when I weighed 290 pounds, I think about how I had no direction and no real reason to get up in the morning. There was nothing about my life that made me jump out of bed and say: "Yeah! Another day!" This was one of the reasons, I realize today, why I became more overweight as the years progressed. I was not happy about much in my life. I had my children and I loved them dearly and certainly wanted to take care of them, but I didn't have anything of my own to look forward to when their basic needs were taken care of. This is what helped foster my poor eating habits and helped hide my unhappiness.

I am talking here about having a purpose in life—something that you have a passion for, that you enjoy doing, and that provides fulfillment. Purpose is the reason you wake up with excitement and anticipation of getting started with your day. This is what will give strength to your actions and motivation to your will. Purpose is what is going to allow you to exert a positive energy and influence wherever you go. I know it does for me, and also for many with whom I speak. We have wasted so many years of our lives obsessing over dieting and food that we allowed that to become our purpose. No wonder we have lost some of our confidence and passion. Now is the time to reclaim your passion and revitalize your life.

You may have many things to do each day—cooking, driving kids to school, mowing the lawn, to name a few—but the actions that will be meaningful to you one year, five years, and ten years from now are those that contribute to your life's purpose. You need to take actions that are making a difference—a meaningful difference in your life, your community, or even the world—no matter how big or small.

It is easy to understand how performing the daily tasks in our lives can lead us to become so consumed with just surviving—paying the bills, raising the kids, maintaining a relationship or a marriage, solving a health problem. Our purpose becomes making it through another week so we can enjoy a day or two on the weekend. This doesn't allow us much time to think about something bigger, something that can make a difference. You don't have to change your career, just define why or for what purpose you do this job. If you are a full-time mother, be sure you realize that at some point this *is* your purpose right now, but that will change when the children are grown. Start to think about what you may be able to do now to prepare yourself for your next role in life or to allow you to be the best at what you are doing now. Can your purpose be to help grow the company you work for to be the best? Can your purpose be to provide a safe community where you live? Can your purpose be "solve world hunger"? Sure, why not?

When you decide on a purpose and it is meaningful to you, then you have motivation, because you have a reason. The more meaningful your purpose is to you, the more motivation it will provide. Remember, I told you that why we do things is just as important, if not more important, than how. After achieving my 130-pound weight loss, I wanted to tell anyone who would listen how I did it. I was just so happy and wanted to share it, maybe even brag a bit, but I quickly learned that actually helping someone else get healthy was even better. This became my purpose. Now I will help anyone in any way I can who wants to lose weight. Every day now I awake with my daily plan, and each action somehow relates to helping others lose weight and get fit. It is very fulfilling to me to help people (you!) succeed with their weight loss. Find what you really get excited about or what you are excited about doing every day in your job, and you will gain that *sense of purpose* in life. When you start living your life for such a purpose, a feeling of self-worth and higher self-esteem will come to you.

A purpose gives you something to focus on that has enough meaning for you that your mission in life becomes much greater than losing weight. Your weight loss and fitness become just a by-product of your main focus—a healthy and active life, one that allows you to realize your full potential. You are starting your new life right now. It is a Self-Improvement through Self-Motivation journey, not a diet or a weight-loss plan. Define a purpose in your life so that you may set yourself up for success when it comes to taking positive and healthy actions.

Living with a strong sense of purpose comes from within and will give you the strength to make the right choices.

Inspiration and Application

Look for sources of inspiration that will instill conviction and determination in your pursuit of better health and fitness. I have shared my story with you and a few stories of others who have changed their lives. Look around in your life, think of those who have overcome great adversity and have gone on to realize their dreams. They are no different from you or me. They did it, I did it, and now it's your turn. Think about times in your life when you accomplished something big, something that made you feel special. It was a great feeling, wasn't it? Can you remember the determination you had then? Conviction and determination are vital to your success and will train your mind to overcome any obstacle that comes your way.

You need a deep-rooted belief that you can be just as successful as the examples from which you are deriving your inspiration. When you are being guided in your daily actions by a strong sense of conviction, you will not be able to be knocked off course, and your determination to realize your goals will make everything that you do an energizing event rather than a chore. Checking off things on the to-do list of your life is incredibly empowering. Think of all the things you do accomplish in life and how great it makes you feel. Relieving your life of this weight-loss burden will be the best accomplishment of all and one that you will be thankful for for many years to come.

Once you have the education as to what foods are unhealthy and what the effects of eating them are, you will have to make a conscious decision to eat in a healthy manner, one bite at a time. If your conviction and determination are strong, there is no way you will make the unhealthy choices. With each step you take in the right direction on this, your Self-Improvement through Self-Motivation journey, your determination and conviction will get stronger. Keep your inspiration in your mind's eye. Realize that each healthy action added to the next healthy action will eventually take shape in your life and the effects will be amazing. Think of the footsteps you want to follow, the examples you want to be led by, so you can do exactly what your role models did.

I realize that this is much easier said than done. In order to do this, you are going to need to develop a sense of motivation that will drive your effort and push every action you take along on this journey.

Motivation

It is so important to know the reasons *why* you wish to lose weight. We discussed this earlier: When you know the "why," the "how" is a lot easier. The most common reasons for wanting to lose weight are for better health, to achieve a higher level of fitness, to feel better, and to look better. These are all good reasons, but they are too general. You want better health, more fitness, to feel more attractive and have more energy? That's great, but what will you do with better health, fitness, shape, and energy? These are the things you must answer for yourself to give you the motivation to succeed. With more energy, will you travel more? Where and when will you travel, and for how long? Will you use your increased energy to engage in more activities: take an educational course, learn how to paint, play with your children (what will you do with them?), get involved with a charity (which one and how often?), take more walks in the park, get a second job? If you want to feel more attractive, what will being more attractive bring you? Will you attract a future spouse, be more attractive to your current spouse, become a model, gain more attention? What activities will you do with your spouse or a new love in your life that you are not doing now? In other words, what will the reasons you have listed bring you or allow you to do that you are not doing now?

In the spaces that follow write down the five things you want to accomplish in life, things you think you can't do now because of your weight. Then write down the reasons why you want to do them or why you must lose weight to do so. If one of your reasons for wanting to lose weight is to have more energy, write it down. Then, if having more energy will allow you to learn to skydive, participate in a local five-mile run for charity, or go downhill skiing, write those down. Keep at this exercise until you come up with five things you want to do and reasons for wanting to lose weight. What will better health allow you to do or bring you? Will it cut your food bill by fifty dollars per week? Will better health allow you to walk without pain, see more clearly, cut your visits to the doctor to only once a year? These must be goals that are real to you, because these are the things that will motivate you. Once you learn these things about yourself, you will see the motivation in black and white. I'm reminded of the child saying, "I want to be something when I grow up," only to become middle-aged and say, "I wish I had been a little more specific." If you want to lose weight, get fit, and be healthy, you must know *why* you desire such things, otherwise you won't know if you are succeeding in your efforts!

Make your list here:

1. _____

  a. _____

  b. _____

  c. _____

2. _____

  a. _____

  b. _____

  c. _____

3. _____

  a. _____

b. _____

c. _____

4. _____

    a. _____

    b. _____

    c. _____

5. _____

    a. _____

    b. _____

    c. _____

Now you have identified five wonderful things you want to do in life and many reasons why losing weight is necessary to get them. These reasons will also coincide with your actions for increasing your healthy thinking, knowing that you are taking steps to make real what is missing in your life. With this action completed, you will begin to see and feel the motivation that will keep you moving toward your desired level of fitness. Remember to read your motivating points and plan your actions for increasing your healthy attitude each day, and over time your foundation for health will grow more stable and therefore will endure for years to come.

Are you curious about what my list of five goals was many years ago when I started on my self-improvement journey? Here it is:

1. **Become Mrs. Missouri**—I knew I would have to get thinner and more fit, and take pride in my appearance again.

2. **Live happily ever after**—Okay, a bit too fairy-tale-ending, but

I am a romantic. I knew that I had to get my moods improved, my attitude soaring, and find love again to be really happy.

3. **Have another baby**—I love children. I was so large that it would have been dangerous to get pregnant again, so I would have to be thinner. I knew this also meant having a husband (see number 2), and I wanted to prove that I could have a healthy pregnancy and not let go and become obese and unhealthy.

4. **Own a successful business**—I was seriously in need of discipline, both professionally and personally, and this made me strive for improvement. Combining my love of business and sales with health and helping others made me very excited and happy.

5. **Help other women better their lives and become more self-assured**—If I could change, then anyone could. It became a motivator for me to be an example to other women whose lives had been torn apart by adultery, obesity, and poor health.

I had other goals: Attend the Oscars, and write a book. Of my seven goals, I have realized five. I am thrilled with my life now, and to think it all started by deciding what I wanted to do and creating a plan of how to go about realizing it. Now it is your turn to do the same.

The best way to instill in yourself a deep-rooted "self-motivation" for this journey is to make it your purpose to improve your life and the lives of your family members and friends. You must decide that being healthy is the most important thing in the world to you because it will enrich not only your life but the lives of all you know and love. Since you now understand the importance of awareness, you should be ready to be more conscious of your choices. This is when self-motivation will be the most important to you. You will acquire this trait slowly over time and strengthen it each time you pass up that cupcake or side of french fries. Each time you successfully jump a hurdle your resolve will be stronger, and the next hurdle will seem much easier to overcome as a result.

You cannot get anywhere without making the effort to arrive at your destination and then taking the actions necessary to get you there. The Road Map I will lay out in Part IV will assist you in changing your negative habits into positive ones and your unhealthy choices into healthy ones.

I believe that motivation is something we can create in our lives. I do not believe that "willpower" is real. An ironclad will that enables you to turn away from unhealthy actions is not something you are born with. It is not something that thin people have and heavy people do not. Willpower is simply the desire to change; it is your determination in action. I know that determination is real and you will replace the pain that your weight has caused you over the years with things that make you feel worthwhile and deserving of the best life has to offer. Replacing the satisfaction or companionship you may have mistaken food for with something that is more lasting will give you much more satisfaction in the long run.

Attitude—Healthy Thinking

The first and most important aspect of being healthy is *thinking* healthy. I'm talking about attitude. You may have heard it before: You must have a good attitude in order to reach all your goals and dreams. Even if you could attain goals without a good attitude, you would feel empty inside without it. There is one very difficult thing about developing a positive and healthy attitude: It can take some time. I can't tell you to get all excited right now because in ten minutes you're going to have the body of your dreams. You know this is not realistic.

It is necessary to realize that changing your thinking will take time. It can be the difference between being self-defeated before you even decide to change and succeeding because you know that you're going to make small changes, one at a time, to overcome a tough mental attitude you may have regarding your weight. Over the years we get discouraged by many failed diet attempts as well as the frustrations that surround our weight problem. This can change our attitude from what used to be one of happiness to one of anger, defeat, and even depression. And we know that the longer we don't change the more often we experience these negative emotions, until one day we live in emotional turmoil. When that happens, the road to emotional stability, happiness, and joy is one that requires actions each day that reinforce positive beliefs and, eventually, impact behavior. Therefore, realize that your change to a healthy attitude will take time, yet will coincide with your change to a healthy and fit body.

This is certainly something you can understand if you have ever been frustrated, discouraged, or angry about being overweight. This is the reason we all need a tune-up when it comes to our thinking and our attitude. I want to give you an exercise to find some basic things to think about that will dramatically change your approach to life. Give yourself sixty days (a reasonable duration) to make the transformation from unhealthy or negative thoughts to empowering and confident beliefs in yourself. But now, take out a pencil and, in the spaces that follow, write down twenty-five very positive aspects about your life today. Maybe you really enjoy gardening, walking, your job, your partner or spouse, the sunshine, the rain, music, shopping, having coffee in the morning, a good friend at work, earning a living, having a house or a place to live that you can call home, your children, a computer, the ability to learn, freedom. Come up with twenty-five specific things you can be happy about or are happy about. If you can't come up with twenty-five items, not to worry; in the next chapter I will help you find a few more.

Write your twenty-five positive things here:

1. _____

2. _____

3. _____

4. _____

5. _____

6. _____

7. _____

8. _____

9. _____

10. _____

11._____

12. _____

13. _____

14. _____

15. _____

16. _____

17. _____

18. _____

19. _____

20. _____

21. _____

22. _____

23. _____

24. _____

25. _____

Now, think of ten or more times in your life when, even as a child, you were very happy. These can be times when you were young when you got good grades, played a musical instrument or your first practical joke, were in love for the first time, got your driver's license, graduated from college, got married, started a new and exciting job, took a vacation, had a child—any event or time of your life that stands out as a happy one. How about when you had your first kiss, performed charity work, painted a picture, saw a movie? What made these times or events special to you? Think about all the little things that made these times enjoyable. What was it about them that brought you happiness? Were you in better physical shape? Did this make you happy because you felt attractive, could find more clothes, or enjoyed shopping? Could you participate in more activities? Did you have a job you really enjoyed? What about the job was enjoyable—the people, the place, the pay?

The reasons that made this time or moment a happy one should be written down on your list. If you listed the same reasons before, use them again here and add why they made you happy. If you enjoyed the people at a job you once had, then write that the people in your job were friendly, or maybe you enjoyed working with a certain co-worker. Perhaps what made you happy about being fit was the ease of shopping for new clothes, or that you felt more attractive, or had more energy, were able to compete in sports or your job—write that down in your list. If you felt joy from a place you had been (maybe a vacation) and the scenery was enjoyable where you were, then write down what about the scenery was enjoyable. No matter how simple a pleasure may seem, put it down. Be sure it is something you can relate to frequently enough so that it can become significant in changing your attitude.

Write the ten most positive memories of your past here:

1. _____

2. _____

3. _____

4. _____

5. _____

6. _____

7. _____

8. _____

9. _____

10. _____

You may not be experiencing these things now, but you did experience them in the past and you know they brought you happiness. You should have a list of things that you are happy about today or that you were once happy about in the past. The reason for these exercises is to recognize what brings you happiness, and to take action to strengthen or fulfill those things on your list that you now know will enable you to have a positive and healthy attitude!

Before you start each day, look over your list and make a conscious decision to take at least one action that will reinforce these positive aspects of your life. If the list contains something from your past that increased your happiness, look at how you can take action today to re-create that same feeling for yourself. Let's say you had a memorable vacation a few years ago, and one of the reasons was because it was warm and sunny. If the sun is not shining today, if it is not warm outside and you can't enjoy that today, go to another point on your list. Maybe you can think about when you had your first child and the joy of having a new life created from your own. Sometimes just remembering something wonderful improves our mood. What can you do today that can give you this same feeling of joy? Hug that child, or write him or her a long letter. I write my children letters all the time and tuck them into their baby books, so that many years from now they will be able to gain insight into me and how much I love them. Perhaps you could spend time with your child (no matter how old), or even just call him or her. How about spending time at a hospital for sick children? Your presence will make them feel better. Any action that will bring you positive fulfillment will raise your emotional level and will be a good thing. Do this each day to eliminate unhealthy thinking and build a lasting foundation of positive, healthy thoughts.

You will see what makes you happy and you will know where to put your energies each day to increase your happiness. This is a slow and sure way to give your attitude a boost. Were we happy as kids because we had no responsibilities? Or was it because we were always playing? We can still do both, just in different ways. Think of this as the game that is your life. The game consists of focusing on what is positive in your life (or what can be) each day by reviewing your list, and then trying to improve upon one or more items each day. Find the good in every aspect of your life, and focus on making those good things better instead of spending time looking at your disappointments. As you and I know, we could go on and on with that list, and it doesn't lead anywhere. That is a self-defeating attitude, and from here on out it must be a thing of your past. Take the actions necessary to create this positive attitude for yourself today and every day and it will help you realize the strength within you. Each day make it a point to improve upon one thing that is already good in your life, as well as experiencing again those things that once made you happy.

Remember, this is a building process. Too many times we try to do too much too fast and our mind as well as our body can't cope with rapid change. The reasons we become overweight are usually the result of habits that have resided with us for some time, and we haven't even been aware of them. Dieting as you did in the past was like trying to stick a finger in the hole in the dam. There is no way such an action could repair the damage, so sooner or later the dam broke and the diet failed. Taking small actions each day to help you improve upon what you are already happy about now, as well as bringing happiness to your life today from memorable events in your past, will give your attitude a positive charge and go a long way toward repairing long-ignored damage.

Rewards

Throughout this book I've assured you that this is not a rigid, restrictive diet plan, but rather a transition to a healthy, energetic way of life. That's not to say the transition is always easy. Along the way we all need some perks to keep our momentum going, some positive reinforcement when things get ho-hum. After seven years of keeping my weight off, certainly there are times when I think about eating pastries, cakes and pies, and pasta with cream sauce. As much as those unhealthy foods may tempt me, I know that I want to continue living the fit, active, and healthy life I am now living. The reason I know this is that the healthy lifestyle gives me many more positive feelings than the unhealthy one ever did. But still, the temptations in life are real and you need a way to defend yourself against them. Be prepared and plan to succeed. My rewards plan will do this for you. I developed this after realizing that by using rewards, my boss was able to get maximum performance out of me and all of the other salespeople. If there was no contest going on, I would apply the minimum amount of effort needed to keep my job. However, if he instituted a contest and there were prizes to be earned, I would kick it into high gear and do whatever was necessary to win the carrots being dangled in front of me.

Since the beginning of "dieting time" we have been trained to associate dieting with deprivation. I will admit to you that I felt deprived every single time I went on a diet. When the all-protein no-carbohydrate diet told me I could not have bread, I thought I would go mad. Just telling me I couldn't have it made me want it more. When I went an entire summer eating only tuna and cantaloupe, I would have killed for a chocolate-chip cookie. I never stopped to realize that getting thinner and healthy was the reward; I just thought I was suffering because I couldn't eat the foods I really wanted.

What made this time different for me, what made it possible for me to change all of these past feelings, was educating myself about what I was doing that was unhealthy for my body and deciding to swear off those things. Sounds like deprivation all over again, doesn't it? Well, this time I added a twist. I rewarded myself for staying away from these unhealthy items or for taking healthy actions.

My biggest "vice" was ice cream—gallon after gallon of it. I didn't just swear off ice cream, because that would be depriving myself. Instead I added something I liked better into the equation. It is important to reward yourself when you meet your goals because it keeps you feeling positive and happy. For example, when I went two weeks without eating any ice cream, I would go and have a full set of nails put on. I came to crave my rewards more than I ever craved ice cream. I think that system is the key not only to how I lost 130 pounds, but also to how I have kept the weight off and will most likely never gain it back. I still treat myself to the pampering, self-indulgent, and soothing rewards now.

There is nothing wrong with wanting to look and feel your best— and rewarding yourself for working to achieve this makes it fun. It made this approach to weight loss and bettering myself different from any diet I had ever gone on—or fallen off of. This time I never went "on" anything, and therefore the day has not arrived when I need to go "off" it. I treat myself well, and I believe in living a full and healthy life. Shouldn't you, as well? After all, aren't you worth it?

Rewards give you the daily encouragement you need to continue doing the actions it takes to be successful with your self-improvement. The quality of the life you can lead from here on out *is* your goal. Becoming fit and healthy grew into a burning desire in my mind because I realized that I wanted to *live.* I have two young children and I really want to watch them grow up. Raising kids is a huge task, filled with a lot of joy, and you get one chance to do it right. And enjoying time with them was certainly a reward I didn't want to miss out on. What are your reasons for wanting to take this path? What are your reasons for wanting to improve your life? Keep them in the forefront of your mind.

As you get used to these perks and rewards of healthy living, you won't want to go back to your old ways. Life today is itself a reward. Give thanks each day for the opportunity to live and grow and change. Every time you apply the principle for healthy living, you are rewarding yourself.

One thing I rarely did as I was first losing my weight was weigh myself, although I could tell when I had lost a substantial amount because my clothes would be bigger. When my clothes seemed a bit bigger, as a special treat or reward, I'd go to a movie or a museum. Usually I went by myself, just to get a break away from the tensions at home and to have some alone time to focus on positive things I wanted to create in my life. After losing enough weight to fit into non-plus-size jeans again, I treated myself to a full hour massage—heaven on earth. The choices of rewards are endless. A reward can be anything you enjoy, that is not food related, of course.

Although a new outfit is a special treat, I don't recommend purchasing a lot of new clothes along the way. Not only might this get you comfortable at a weight that is short of your goal, but you will also be wasting money on clothes that will be too big once you've lost more weight. Try purchasing accessories to revitalize an outfit or an item that will be easier to take in than a dress or suit. This is not to say you shouldn't buy a special outfit or a few new things, but don't do the whole new wardrobe until you have reached your goal.

My rewards helped instill the motivation I needed to continue each step of the way. I was beginning to feel like a woman again. I wasn't just a mom anymore or someone's discarded wife. It was great to feel alive, worthwhile, and vibrant—for the first time in years!

In order to earn rewards, you need to know what you are rewarding yourself for. Establish goals for yourself, both long- and short-term goals. Then create a list of things you would want as a reward or treat once you meet that goal. I have recommended that people buy tickets to a concert or event coming to town in a month or so; if you don't meet the goals you've set by then, you don't go. You have to give the tickets away. Earn the treat or don't get it. Apply the knowledge that you have gotten or you don't earn a reward. It is that easy.

When using a rewards system, you are setting yourself up for success. You are taking the control of your life back, not putting yourself on some diet that will only doom you to failure. I still use this system and I am still not dieting today. Rewards are necessary in all we do. When I am done writing, responding to E-mails, or with a day of telephone calls, I will spend time with the children, go somewhere on the weekend for the day, or just see a movie—my rewards for completing the tasks at hand. I use my rewards so I'm always looking forward to accomplishing a chore. This really can change your perspective. Setting goals and laying out a plan outlining how you are going to achieve them is the only way to realize the life that awaits you.

It is important that you identify your "vice" and use the rewards plan to help you "bust" it. We will deal with this more in Level II of your actions.

Make your goal sheet look something like this:

WEEK 1: No _____ (Ice cream was mine.)

WEEK 2: No _____ (Ice cream again.)

    Reward: _____ (Manicure was mine.)

WEEK 3: Walk 20 minutes 3 times, no _____

WEEK 4: Walk 25 minutes 3 times, no _____

    Reward: _____ (Haircut and style for me.)

3-month goal: _____ (Reward here.)

6-month goal: _____ (Reward here.)

1-year goal: _____ (Reward here.)

Review after each week, and update each month. Part IV: "The Road Map to Weight Loss and Fitness" will help you pinpoint specific actions you need to take and changes you need to make. Reward yourself along the way as you master each level.

By the end of six weeks, you will definitely be feeling better about yourself, your health will be improving, and you will most likely be at least ten pounds thinner. You will be looking better—with your new nails and maybe a new hairdo—and you will possibly possess some new knowledge found in an exhibit at a local museum. I guarantee that people will ask what you have done differently. The one answer you will *not* give is "I have been dieting." Never again will that be your answer. No, you are changing your life. You will most likely have more energy and be feeling proud of yourself for reaching your goals. You will have lost weight and you will find that it seemed so easy this time. You weren't counting calories, you weren't watching what food groups you were combining. You were simply eating healthy foods and drinking more water. It is that easy. You will be doing small "baby step" actions that over time lead to huge changes.

It is important that you identify what will work for you as rewards. They are, of course, different for each person. What do you like about how you look today? Pretty eyes, a nice smile, a good complexion? Are there things that could stand improvement? What about your hair? Have you let it go as well as your body? While it may take time to get your body back to a normal weight, you can fix your hair right now. You can buy a new shade of lipstick today. Manicures, pedicures, and facials are a wonderful treat. You deserve to spend a little time and a little money on yourself. I promise you that doing this will make you feel so revived, like a new woman. Massages and body polishing are also great treats. Sure, the thought of a stranger seeing you practically naked is frightening. After you have lost twenty-five or fifty pounds, however, you won't mind. Buy some scented candles. Burning them at night gives such a nice peaceful scent around the house and creates the same mood. A bouquet of fresh flowers on your kitchen or dining-room table will make you feel special. How about buying a new CD that is a relaxing New Age sound? Eat healthfully for a month and treat yourself to the music that you will be in heaven with. You could even listen to it while you take a bath. Rewards don't have to cost money; you can sightsee a grand neighborhood in your hometown, visit a longtime friend, draw a picture, organize your photos into albums, sunbathe, or nap in the middle of the day!

The key to this rewards system is to remember that you may do these things if—and only if—you earn them. By that I mean successfully meeting the goal you placed on the particular reward. Make your goal a worthwhile and meaningful one that you can be proud of, and your reward will be just the—uh—icing on the cake? Well, a great added bonus!

PART IV

The Road Map to Weight Loss and Fitness

The F~~oo~~d HEALTH Pyramid

I call the plan for action outlined here the Road Map. It will change the way you approach your weight loss. It is designed to allow you to make easy, gradual changes that will last and keep you moving toward the lifestyle you desire. Remember that most diet plans or programs are laid out in a way that forces you to overhaul your daily actions in order to implement their plan. For many years, plans have been sold to us that I can sum up for you in one sentence: Cut down on your total daily calorie intake and start exercising each day. That's everything you need to do to get healthy and fit. If it's that simple, why have we not succeeded? Why does the problem keep getting worse? As I stated before, it's because the changes necessary to do this are overwhelming, which makes us feel that the task at hand is just too huge for us to handle and therefore we give up. That is why the plan laid out for you here, as you will notice, is gradual and easy to follow.

If you have less than fifty pounds to lose, you may not be experiencing the same emotions as those who have one hundred or more, but you still feel that the task is great and success has eluded you before. Needless to say, you will still benefit from taking the same actions I have outlined here. Even the last ten pounds can seem overwhelming to the person who has been trying to lose them for years. Depending on where you are in your weight-loss and fitness level, you can decide at which step you may want to begin. In other words, if you are just beginning, then you will want to start at Level I. In contrast, if you have lost forty pounds and need to lose your last twenty, then you may be able to accomplish the first couple of levels without much effort, or you may already be living at those levels so you'll be able to proceed directly to higher levels.

Before getting into the step-by-step plan, let's go over *the* fundamental guideline for healthy living. If you have been overweight your entire life and think that you were taught and actually use healthy eating habits, you may want to go to a physician who specializes in obesity. Get checked out and make sure that you are not suffering from any illnesses. Tell your physician you don't want to be put on a diet but that you want the facts about what is good for you and your health. While you're at it, ask why the government's food pyramid recommends so many starches, and why the new body mass index (BMI) is set up in a way that defines most of us as obese. They push starches on us; we gain more weight. Then they call us fat and tell us it's our fault.

The food pyramid as it exists is outdated and wrong. This is because the base of the pyramid consists of starches or carbohydrates, recommending so many servings of them that it is little wonder 55 percent of Americans are overweight. I believe we were not given a pyramid model that would lead to optimal health. Getting a visual picture of what's most important when it comes to what you eat and drink will help you remember what you should be eating or drinking the most, as well as the least. Refer to my pyramid often. Stick to the basics—those things that make a strong foundation for good health and, ultimately, fitness. And because we are changing the way it looks, don't view it as a food pyramid, but as a *health pyramid.* This health pyramid should be the cornerstone of your diet. Don't get ahead of yourself here; this is what your health pyramid will be when you are fit, not today when you decide to get fit and are just starting your journey. Just like Rome, building it will take time.

Water: The Number-One Compound for Health

The first and most important substance you ingest should be water. Many may disagree with me on this, but I believe the majority of what we consume should be water. Not based on weight or calories, but based on volume. Water has more benefits for our bodies than any other substance. After all, what are we largely made up of? Water!

Think of water as flushing and eliminating toxins out of your body. All the additives and chemicals that are put in, added to, or sprayed on foods, and all the contaminants that are in the air we breathe—in the home and outside—are more easily eliminated with adequate water consumption. Water cleanses, clears, purifies, and rinses your body's cells, glands, organs, and systems. Water will also help maintain blood pressure as well as your body temperature. All the systems of your body will experience more optimal function with proper hydration. It has been estimated that 75 percent of Americans are not drinking enough water. That means that the majority of us are experiencing dehydration to some degree. Any other fluids that may be made up of mostly water don't count toward your daily intake because they do not have the same benefit as just plain water. It's not news that we all need at least eight glasses of water each day. If you are sixty-five pounds or more overweight, chances are you need ten. Water is the foundation for good health. Make carrying a water bottle your habit, something you can't go anywhere without. Never leave home without it! I have a water bottle with me at all times.

Exercise—Get Moving!

The next most important aspect of weight loss and fitness is incorporating some form of extra physical activity into your daily life. Exercise as we know it has become something of a chore because of our sedentary lifestyles. With the advent of machines that do most of the work that once required our physical labor, we do not expend the same number of calories as a society that we once did. In order to make up for this, we need to perform some form of movement above and beyond our normal daily activities. Exercise is the next block on your health pyramid for many good reasons.

Just as water provides oxygen to your cells and systems of your body, so too does exercise. Performing some form of exercise that increases your heart rate and your respiratory rate (breathing) will increase the flow of freshly oxygenated blood to all parts of your body. This means more oxygen to the brain to stimulate healthy thinking, too! Remember that another of the body's most important elements for healthy function is oxygen. If your body has been overweight for any length of time, you probably are not getting enough oxygen to the cells, organs, and systems in your body. Exercise can help do that for you. Being overweight, your body is probably not functioning at its full potential.

Exercise increases the strength of the heart and lungs, which will give you more energy and the ability to perform more activities. If one of your reasons for wanting to lose weight is increased energy (in order to spend more time with your kids, travel, etc.), then exercise is a must. I hear women tell me that they are too tired to exercise, and it is difficult to do something when they don't have the energy. This is more of a mental barrier than a physical one. I can attest to the fact that my energy levels have increased exponentially now that I exercise at least three times a week, and usually five. If you want to feel more awake, feel more energy, and have more creative thoughts, exercise will provide that for you. Maybe you have heard of "runner's high"? This is the result of two chemicals that are released in the body called endorphins and enkephalins. They are responsible for giving us that feeling of euphoria. So exercise will improve your attitude as well because of the release of these chemicals. What an amazing fact that we have all the antidepressants and mood stimulants we need inside of us, just waiting for us to get moving so that we can utilize them.

There are many stories of people who have been diagnosed with a disease who have changed their lifestyle to include exercise and have gone on to beat their ailment or at least substantially improve their quality of life and their prognosis. Remember, they don't call obesity the second leading cause of preventable death in America for nothing. Exercise will put you on the path to the life of fitness and health that you desire and keep you firmly planted on the path of Self-Improvement through Self-Motivation. *If you feel you don't have the energy to exercise, you really don't have the energy not to exercise.*

As you embark on the road to health and fitness, there will certainly be days when you feel you have ruined your progress by splurging on an unhealthy food or succumbing to fast food. Be realistic and anticipate that this may happen, even when you have been so good as to avoid such actions. Not to worry. If and when you have developed a daily habit of doing some form of exercise, you can put in an extra few minutes to make up for any "damage" you feel you may have done. In other words, if you feel you have "cheated" on your healthy eating plan, exercise can compensate for the added calories you may have taken in. This does not give you license to eat what you want because you know you will be burning some of the calories off later; that would give you no net weight loss at all, and perhaps you would gain weight (although minimal, it can add up). But it is to say that exercise can be somewhat of a "safety net" as you are developing consistent habits that parallel a healthy and fit body.

A last point about the importance of exercise: I have found that many of my readers are older than thirty-five years of age, and they believe it is more difficult to lose weight as they get older. From my experience, they are right and at the same time they are wrong. They are right because the years of habits that are a part of their daily lives make it harder to change, and the body's metabolism slows down as we age. They are wrong because they can overcome this mental barrier and because there are ways to get the metabolism going again. Increasing the amount of physical activity each day will provide that increased metabolism. If you put more demands on your body each day by exercising, you will be training your body to be prepared for the next time you do such activity. Therefore you will give your metabolism a boost that can eventually become permanent with such continued daily actions.

One of the things I regret I did not do for the first six months of my new lifestyle was exercise. I lost a lot of weight without exercise, so I know that only eating right can make a significant change to your body. Yet in retrospect, I may have not been able to handle the considerable change to my lifestyle had I tried to exercise immediately after deciding to embark on my path of self-improvement. I put exercise after water as the next most important aspect of building a healthy lifestyle because I truly believe that my weight loss has been maintained, along with my increased energy level, more positive attitude, and decreased level of stress, with consistent and regular exercise.

When I first started exercising, I took an aerobics class three times a week. I went at my own pace and didn't try to keep up with my already fit classmates. I recommend doing the same if you are able. If you are not, start walking twenty minutes a day. A reader was 100 pounds overweight and her doctor told her she "was fat, would always be fat." She was having trouble walking so he handed her a cane. She started walking a little bit each day and is now ninety pounds lighter and training for a marathon. As for the cane, she keeps that nearby to "knock things off of a high shelf."

I am amazed when I hear the "eight minutes in the morning," "five minutes a day," or "ten minutes three times a week" pitches for various diet or exercise plans. If the body I have today could have been achieved in five minutes a day or maintained by exercising for a few minutes in the morning, trust me, I would know about it, would have tried it, and would be doing it. As much as I love the results I get from exercise, let's face it, a lot of time is spent going to and from the gym and at the gym. If there was an easier way or a shortcut, I would be all for it, but to date I haven't found it.

My "love" of exercise is an acquired trait. I started with my few aerobics classes and gained the strength and confidence to move to the next level. My typical exercise regimen today is sixty minutes five days a week of cardiovascular exercise, such as the treadmill or elliptical machine, and forty-five minutes of weight training three days a week. I also strive to take an aerobics class on Saturday mornings. Exercise has become a routine part of my life.

Fruits and Vegetables:
Vitamin and Mineral Rich

With oxygen being so essential to good health, it is easy to conclude that fruits and vegetables, which are high in water content and therefore oxygen, are healthy. There are many reasons why fruit is the next building block for good health, but first and foremost is the fact that fruits have high levels of water, vitamins, and fiber. With so much importance put on water, it's an added bonus to have a snack that not only tastes good, but also has a high water content. Add the vitamin content of fruit and you've got a great healthy choice.

Some may argue that because fruits contain a significant amount of sugar, fruit consumption should be limited. I strongly disagree. I can't imagine that a food so natural, a food that comes from Mother Nature and has not been altered by processing, additives, preservatives, and the chemicals so many other foods contain can be harmful to you, your weight, or your health. I call it "God's sugar": If He made it, feel free to consume it. Of course, like all foods, fruits should be consumed in moderation. Too much of any food is not healthy.

I understand that today most fruits are sprayed with chemicals to protect them from pesky varmints and insects, so be sure to wash your fruit before eating it.

Most vegetables are also water based. They contain a beneficial amount of vitamins *and* minerals, as well as high fiber. One of the more common deadly diseases today is colon cancer. Many reports recommend more fiber for a healthier colon and a healthier body overall. Most people's fiber consumption has dropped off substantially over the past decades. I believe this is because our fruit and vegetable intake has dropped. I don't see many fast-food restaurants serving spinach, broccoli, or asparagus. I've never known anyone to be overweight because they were consuming too many carrots or salads. I think of salads and vegetables as human body cleansers. Fruits and vegetables are the most-used food group for me now, and they were during my weight loss. I ate a veggie sandwich for lunch every day for months. Boring? Perhaps. Healthy? You bet! If I am going to a party, I bring a vegetable tray. This way I know there will be something healthy to snack on. Think of fiber as a cleanser of your colon, which is where many toxins lurk and can be eliminated. Eating lots of vegetables will help ensure a healthy colon. You will be getting the proper daily intake of vitamins and minerals that are so important to good health. Vegetables translate into better digestion and organ function, healthy cells, and an overall happier body. I recommend finding a few vegetables you enjoy and sticking with them. For a list of recommended fruits and vegetables, refer to the "Grocery List" on pages 267–268.

Meats, Fish, and Other Proteins: Strength Builders

As you probably know, protein is used by the body to build muscle. Protein will provide your body with the amino acids and some of the minerals needed for healthy functioning. Unlike fat or carbohydrates, though, protein, if it's not needed, is not stored in your body to be used later. This means you can have a high-protein meal, feel full, get needed nutrition, and not necessarily gain weight. This is not an endorsement for eating only proteins, but it is to say that putting lean proteins ahead of carbohydrates and starches is going to be of great benefit when it comes to losing weight.

Protein is often called the "building block" of a healthy body. The body uses protein to repair and rebuild. Protein can be found in your muscles, hair, skin, nails—all things that I want looking great! Your enzymes, hormones, and immune system all require protein to function optimally.

If you eat a diet low in protein, your body is not able to produce the amino acids it needs to function. When this happens, the body starts to break down muscle to compensate for the lack of protein. The reason you do not want this to happen is that it slows down your metabolism. Your metabolism is what burns calories and fat. Make sure to eat healthy protein throughout the day. I keep hard-boiled eggs in the fridge and often grab one and eat only the egg white, which has only fifteen calories and tons of protein—the perfect snack. For a detailed list of healthy protein sources, refer to the "Grocery List" on pages 267–268.

Carbohydrates and Starches: Use It or You *Won't* Lose It

Carbohydrates are considered one of the most important parts of a healthy diet. We all need a source of energy to carry out our movements, activities, exercises, and more. Every cell, organ, and system in our body requires a source of energy in order to function—our heart to beat, our bowels to function, our legs to move, our minds to think, and so on. Carbohydrates are the sugars we use for this energy. Breads, pastas, candy, sodas, wines, beer, fruits—all have a form of carbohydrates. Carbohydrates are certainly important when looked at from this perspective. Yet it is also important to remember that if you do not use the carbohydrates and starches you consume, your body will store them for future use. And if you consume too much, your body will store carbohydrates as fat. (My homeless man should have shouted, "Girl, you got too much carbohydrates in you!")

We hear people mention "good carbs" and "bad carbs" and offer us their opinion on which is better for us. When you eat carbohydrates, the body digests them and converts them into glucose (our blood's sugar). They then enter the bloodstream to be burned as energy.

Imagine what happens when you eat a meal that is high in carbohydrates, such as a bagel with jam and fruit juice or a plate of pasta with tomato sauce. Your body goes into overdrive converting all of this into glucose for energy to be burned immediately. That is not bad, except for the fact that what you are not burning now is "stored energy"—or, as we lovingly call it, fat!

My husband, Dr. Patrick Havey, tells me that "fats burn best in a flame of carbohydrates" and therefore carbohydrates are best eaten before working out. The fat-burning process has to be started with some carbohydrates (the flame), and of course to get this fire going and keep it going, it is necessary to exercise by doing some form of sustained physical activity (fifteen minutes or more at a time). In order to create this flame a small amount of carbohydrate is needed—a piece of fruit is a good example.

Carbohydrates are divided into two groups: simple carbohydrates and complex carbohydrates. *Simple carbohydrates,* sometimes called simple sugars, include fructose (fruit sugar), sucrose (table sugar), and lactose (milk sugar), as well as several others. Fruits are one of the richest natural sources of simple carbohydrates. *Complex carbohydrates* are also made up of sugars, but the sugar molecules are strung together to form longer, more complex chains. Complex carbohydrates include fiber and starches. Foods rich in complex carbohydrates include vegetables, whole grains, peas, and beans.

Fruits contain natural sugars, fiber, and vitamins. The best form of starch is a baked potato. If you can eat a potato raw, even better. Again, the rule of thumb here is to eat things that are straight from nature, not processed or broken down into another form. Cereal is the best example of a food that is high in sugar and broken down from natural (and many not-so-natural) sources. Cereals are often marketed as healthy products because they are touted as having essential vitamins and minerals. However, you will do yourself far more harm than good by consuming most cereals on the market today. This is because the majority of them are sugar laden. If you choose a cereal, make it one low in sugar content (less than ten grams per serving) and high in fiber. Personally, I like Bob's Red Mill Muesli cereal. Add to it vegetable protein, some wheat bran, and fresh berries and then you've got yourself a true "Breakfast of Champions."

Here is what your health pyramid looks like. Remember, you are building this pyramid, as opposed to starting to live by it tomorrow. When your pyramid is built, it will be next to impossible to knock it down, push it over, move it, or destroy it, so long as your positive actions become strong habits and your habits have created a strong and healthy you. Let's start taking action.

Food Guide Pyramid
A Guide to Daily Food Choices

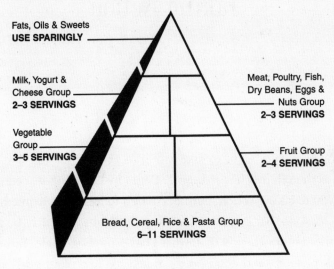

Fats, Oils & Sweets
USE SPARINGLY

Milk, Yogurt &
Cheese Group
2–3 SERVINGS

Vegetable
Group
3–5 SERVINGS

Meat, Poultry, Fish,
Dry Beans, Eggs &
Nuts Group
2–3 SERVINGS

Fruit Group
2–4 SERVINGS

Bread, Cereal, Rice & Pasta Group
6–11 SERVINGS

Source: U.S. Department of Agriculture

The Health Pyramid by Julia

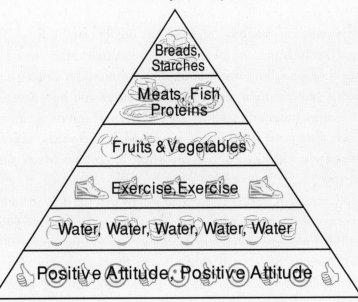

Breads,
Starches

Meats, Fish
Proteins

Fruits & Vegetables

Exercise, Exercise

Water, Water, Water, Water, Water

Positive Attitude, Positive Attitude

Taking Action

Remember as you begin to take action to get fit that you don't want to feel as though much is changing. Begin by changing just enough to know you're taking action, but not enough to feel overwhelmed. If you have a lifestyle that consists of fairly good habits, you may be able to move ahead more quickly than what I have suggested here. Either way, don't skip a step, and don't do too much too fast. Your goals are significant, and it's worth taking the time to do this right. While to some my 130-pound weight loss may seem to have occurred at a very fast pace, it didn't. I lost 130 pounds in fifteen months—that averages out to 8 pounds a month, 2 pounds a week, and mere ounces a day.

To the naysayers who look at these actions and believe they won't work because they are too simple as they do not count calories, factor in food combinations, or calculate body mass index, they are right. If you believe something won't work, then it won't. But before you discard this easy program, don't forget the times you may have failed with another program that addressed all of these complicated points. We have gotten too smart for our own good. Keep to these simple actions and you will succeed. It's only when things become too complicated that giving up becomes a much easier solution to our efforts. When you reach a level of fitness that is now familiar only to a smaller percentage of the population, then you can begin to immerse yourself in stricter programs and details. For now, let's keep it simple.

The "perfect body" still eludes me; I guess I am not obsessing enough about food. I am in good shape and look and feel wonderful. I'm guessing that most of us would be happy to be in good health and

good shape, and are not looking to become supermodels or professional athletes. So remember: Keep it simple.

I have designed a lifestyle approach in nine levels. Each level
should be mastered at your own pace. Do not move on to the next
level until you feel confident about your new lifestyle change. You are
not in a race with anyone. There is no need to rush; it is more important to get it right this time. There will not be a prize handed out
to the person who loses the most weight the fastest. You do not need
to hold up a newspaper and have your picture taken with it to signal
the start of your diet. Master this level before taking on more change.
Remember, doing it this way will help you not to be overwhelmed
and not to feel that you just can't lose the weight. You can and you
will—one step at a time. It may take one person a week to master a
particular level, and for another it could be months. This is your journey. Do it the right way for you to achieve permanent change. As you
begin your journey, it is important to check with your health-care
provider. It is important for him or her to agree with what you are
embarking on and to be aware of anything new you are doing. Get
your doctor's okay and blessing before commencing. I remember
when I told my doctor that I was finally ready to change. He hugged
me, prayed with me, and wished me luck.

LEVEL I
Getting Started

At this point you have completed your exercise for a healthy attitude. You have taken the time to list the reasons why you want to be fit, and therefore you realize what you will do with more fitness, more energy, and better health. Start today by reviewing your lists and planning actions to create more fulfillment in your life. Just an extra action or two each day will lift your spirits and enforce your positive thinking. If you have to revise your list in order to be sure you have things that are meaningful to you, please do. Make the next few days ones you use to think about the life you will have without the extra weight, being at the level of fitness you desire. Each day review your list and plan your actions, take the time to picture the life you will have, and include your motivating points, as if they are real to you today. These first few days are vital to your weight-loss success. By taking these simple actions each day, you will be creating a new picture of your life—of how you want it to be!

If you don't know where you're going, you won't know if you are getting any closer, or whether you've arrived.

This first week you are actually creating a picture of the life you will be living at the weight you desire. What will you be doing differently on a daily basis? Picture yourself at this weight and the things you will be doing differently. Define in your mind the actions you will be doing or doing better, on a daily basis. Author Mark Victor Hansen (*Chicken Soup for the Soul*) describes "visualization as realization" in his books. Before anything becomes reality it must first be a thought. Your reality of the life you desire must be a very clear thought before it becomes real. Otherwise you won't know if you're there, because you won't know where you're going. Provide yourself with details about your life's picture. See yourself in that picture, feel yourself there—the sounds, the smells, the colors of your picture. This will reinforce the reasons why you want to be fit. The motivation becomes real, your desire becomes real. We all complain about being sick and tired of being overweight. The pain of being overweight overshadows what we desire in a life of health and fitness. You need reasons other than just being tired of the extra weight, or being sick of feeling unattractive. What is the opposite of being overweight and unhappy? Being fit, happy, attractive, confident, more productive, more energetic? Can you even imagine yourself living that life? If you have been overweight for your entire life, this week may be the most difficult for you. How do you imagine something you have never known?

Picture what you will be doing on a day that consists of having these qualities you long for. Are you waking up with more energy to exercise, traveling to the mountains with your children, going hiking, spending the evening walking in the park, shopping in a mall for your favorite clothes, going on a date with a new love in your life, working hard and earning that job promotion, using your time helping a charity? Heck, for some of us just being able to do the simple things like getting out of the bathtub without difficulty or being able to walk without the aid of a cane is hard to imagine. But you must imagine it, in order to allow it to become real. You must imagine it to be able to grow your dream into an action and then into a habit and a way of life.

Identify yourself in this picture having the qualities that losing weight will bring you. Make this the picture of your daily life that you strive for—the life you aim to create as a result of losing weight. Each morning when you wake up, read your list of reasons to be happy today, and plan an action for the day to experience one or more items on your list. Also, read your motivation and to-do list, and be sure to picture yourself having the things you desire that will come as a result of your weight-loss efforts. These are important actions to build the foundation for an attitude of health and fitness.

The next action to take during your first week is an easy one. Look at the fluids you consume on a regular basis that aren't water: any soft drinks, juices, or any drink that has a high amount of sugar, even diet sodas or diet drinks. Replace them with water one by one. Buy yourself a water bottle, preferably a sixteen-ounce plastic bottle that you will carry with you *all the time.* For stylish people, handbag designers are even catching on. You can buy a fancy holder for your bottle now. Instead of drinking anything else, unless it's your morning cup of coffee or tea (with no sugars, syrups, or chocolate added), drink water. I even keep a water bottle on my nightstand for times when I may be thirsty during the night or upon waking. Many times when I feel that I may be hungry or want something to eat I drink water, only to realize that I was simply thirsty.

As explained earlier, consuming enough water will give your body a boost in its ability to eliminate extra, unwanted weight. I would even recommend buying a water filter to be sure your water is of good quality. There are many brands available and many stores that carry them. You will feel good knowing that you're drinking good, clean water. You will also gain a sense of commitment and responsibility by making a small investment in a filter. Each time you see your filter you will know that you're doing your body good.

Water is the only change you need to make in your diet for the first week. If you could only see the letters I get from readers telling me how shocked and amazed they are that, after only two weeks of breaking their sugar-drink addiction, they have lost seven, eight, or even ten pounds. They lost that amount of weight without changing anything else. Is that enough incentive for you to do this and master Level I? I hope so.

HERE IS A REVIEW OF YOUR ACTIONS FOR LEVEL I:

1. Review your list of positive things in your life and what you can do to improve at least one each day. Each day review the reasons why you want to lose weight, revising or adding to the list as necessary. Picture your life as you will be living it as a fit and healthy person.
2. Buy a filter for your water, and also buy a sixteen-ounce water bottle. Carry your water bottle with you at all times, and substitute water for any other fluids you have been drinking. You can drink a cup of coffee or tea each day (no gourmet coffees, no sugars added, but low-cal sweeteners), and a glass of skim milk if necessary, but be sure to consume at least three sixteen-ounce bottles of water each day.

LEVEL II
Replacing the Bad with the Good: "Vice Busting"

Now that you have put time and energy into making your vision of your new life clear and you have taken the basic action of drinking plenty of water each day, it is time to make some changes regarding your diet. Take a look at the items or types of foods you consume on a regular basis that you could honestly say are unhealthy and keeping weight on you. It's time to identify the worst habit you have, isolate it from your routine, and work on eliminating it from your new lifestyle. Choose from the items you snack on between meals. Do you eat potato chips, pizza, chocolate, cereal, candy, cakes, or cookies? Identify the one food or type of food you consume on a regular basis that is contributing to your extra weight. If you have an afternoon snack that is high in sugar or fat, like cookies, chips, or white bread, it's time to replace it with something healthy and tasty. You do not need to reinvent the wheel or change your routine; you just need to change what you are choosing to nibble on. The surveys I have received from thousands of dieters indicate that there are certain foods we seem to have a weakness for that keep us from losing weight. In order to get rid of these bad habits, we need to replace this item with something else so we don't feel denied. What could be as good as those items? you ask. How about a piece of fruit? Fruit is not only healthy, with its high water, vitamin, and fiber content, but also tastes good. Fruit is a source of natural sugars, so it will satisfy your sweet tooth while providing sound nutrition. I used carrots to replace my unhealthy snacks, and carried with me a small bag of bite-size carrots to snack on. If you can find any fruit or vegetable that you enjoy, that you can carry with you to work or at home, start to use it as a substitute for all the unhealthy snacks or one unhealthy food "vice" you may have. If you like oranges or apples, buy a bag of either, or both, that will last you the week. Be sure to keep one or two on hand when you are at work or away from your home. If you have to carry your fruit in your purse, try grapes or cut up an orange and put it in a plastic bag. You can also choose carrots or raisins as your substitute, as well as most items that you will find in the fruit and vegetable section of your supermarket. Choose a few to allow you the variety, but keep it simple, and be sure to keep your items available. This is the only added action for the week. Remember, this is designed to allow you to change at a pace that is manageable. You need not starve—that will do you no good. If you feel as though you could eat nonstop and binge, fine. Do so, but eat something healthy like raisins, carrots, or apples. Trust me, this bingeing won't go on for long.

As an aside, I would like to suggest that you affirm your commitment to succeeding by taking all of the unhealthy snacks (the cookies, crackers, candies, or any other high-sugar treats you eat often) you have in your cabinets or refrigerator and either throwing them out or giving them to a homeless shelter. Most of the people I have seen at the Salvation Army or soup kitchens are not struggling with having "too much food in them." They have bigger problems and could use some assistance. This will be good for you and for them!

HERE IS A REVIEW OF YOUR ACTIONS FOR LEVEL II:

1. Review and revise your list of positive things about your life, as well as your motivating reasons for getting fit.
2. Carry your water bottle with you at all times.
3. Repace your biggest "vice snacks" with healthy food—fruits or vegetables.
4. Use your rewards plan to help you "bust" your "vice."

Do not move on to Level III until you have mastered Level II as well as continuing to adhere to the changes you made in Level I.

Level III
Starting Some Form of Exercise

Adding some form of physical activity to your daily actions will be a great boost to your weight-loss efforts. This week you must plan to implement some form of exercise each day, which will help you burn more calories than you do now. Make your activity something easy to get started doing, something you feel you can handle. Plan what you will do and when. Taking a walk each day during your lunch hour at work (be sure to bring your sneakers) is one example that is easy to do. Start with fifteen minutes of exercise each day. If you would like to join a gym, or use at-home equipment, do so with the intention of doing no more than fifteen minutes of exercise a day. If you are tempted to jump in with both feet because your determination is high, don't. Do just enough to know you have put in the effort, but not so much that you feel run-down and unable or unwilling to exercise again tomorrow. The idea here is to develop the habit of exercising, and to get in a daily routine that will be lasting. If you don't want to use your lunch hour at work, you could use a ten-minute break and walk the stairs in your building. Be sure this is not too strenuous, and if it is, turn to walking.

Moving will help you think, give you more ideas, help clean your body of toxins, and help accelerate your elimination of unwanted weight. Any form of extra movement each day will help revitalize your body and mind. If you feel you don't have the energy to do any form of exercise, realize that you must exercise (even if it's just for five or ten minutes) to acquire the energy you need to do the things you are missing out on in life, not just to lose weight. Think of the weight loss as a great bonus of healthy living. This thought will help to cement the idea that a healthy lifestyle is meant to last long past the duration of the "diet du jour," which is the "old" way of thinking. A healthy lifestyle needs to become ingrained in your mind and be second nature to you. Then and only then will you lose the weight you desire, and keep it off for the rest of your life.

One of the most difficult things to do, especially if you have a substantial amount of weight to lose, is take up exercise. The hesitation we feel at having to go to a gym to use the machines or partake in an aerobics class because we are self-conscious about our weight is certainly a barrier that must be overcome. If you are feeling this way, one solution is to do your exercise on your own. I suggest walking because it's easy to do, it can be done almost anywhere, and it does not require buying expensive gym memberships or equipment, just the right walking shoes. The time for joining a gym or purchasing an at-home piece of exercise equipment is after you have developed a daily habit of exercising for some time. This will be an action to look forward to for the future. Remember, I didn't exercise for the first six months of my path to fitness. It was only after I had developed good habits for an extended period of time that I became comfortable participating in an aerobics class three times a week. At this point I knew I might get discouraged with my physical ability (or lack thereof), but this wouldn't cause me to give up on my goal because I had already come a long way. In the end I was able to overcome my inabilities because of my added determination and confidence. In time, you will become more confident in your abilities than you are today. It just takes time and persistence. Therefore, be sure that each day you commit to doing some form of added physical activity for fifteen minutes. Of course, before embarking on any exercise plan you may want to consult your doctor to make sure that you have no hidden health issues that may be affected by a particular form of exercise.

As you start to exercise each day, it may also help to find a partner or even a group to exercise with. If others also desire to improve their health, you can motivate each other. Perhaps you know someone who is already on her way to achieving her goals and has made progress who would like your company. You'd be surprised at how many people would love to help someone starting out because they know the difficulty of getting into the habit and getting over the hump during the first few weeks of exercising. You will also be supporting their efforts, because you will make them feel as though they are a source of inspiration for you. We all need a support system to help us stay focused on our goals, especially during those days when other stresses may be getting us down or keeping us from taking action. Don't feel that you're not worthy of talking with or hanging out with an associate or acquaintance who is more fit than you. Other people on the same path will respect you for your interest and your dedication to getting fit, and they will be glad to help.

Varying your routine may help keep your interest. Try something different on one weekend day, like walking in a museum, or in a park, or in the mall in the morning while you window-shop. How about taking the kids with you? Make it fun, and be sure to give yourself a day of rest each week to reflect on your progress. I usually do not work out on Sunday; I like to make that my family day.

HERE IS A REVIEW OF YOUR ACTIONS FOR LEVEL III:

1. Review your positive and motivational points each day.
2. Drink lots of water every day.
3. Substitute fruits or vegetables as snacks or between meals.
4. Do some form of exercise for fifteen minutes each day.

Stick to these actions each day for the first few weeks. Make it simple and easy for yourself in order to develop these habits for a good foundation for building health and losing weight. Do not move on to Level IV until you have mastered each of the points in the previous levels. Why take on more change until you are 100 percent totally committed to applying the changes that you have already been learning? When you are ready, you will have Levels I, II, and III ingrained in you and they will be second nature. Take some extra time if you need to, and do not assume more change until you are securely on the path of self-improvement.

LEVEL IV
Journal/Diary

Continue doing the same actions you have started for your first few weeks. Let your body and mind feel the changes you have initiated. With these changes alone you will experience a sense of better health—mentally and physically. It is important that you understand your thoughts and feelings. In this level I want you to focus on getting to know yourself better. Buy a notebook or diary, keep it with you as often as possible, and use it to write down ideas, memories, thoughts—anything that comes to mind. The only rule or guideline here is that you do not write about food. Not about how much you wanted to eat or how much you did eat. Think of it this way: If an archaeologist were to find your journal a hundred years from now and it contained information on how many grams of this or calories of that you ate, he or she would think you were a science experiment, not a person! Let this journal be a testament to you, who you are and what you want out of life. Use it to elaborate on the discoveries you made earlier in the book.

Besides getting to know yourself better in this level, be sure you are getting adequate water intake, cutting out "vice" foods, and getting the appropriate amount of exercise. Make this a week you can look back on with a feeling of success because you remained committed to your healthy actions. Make it a week when you will make the extra effort to adhere completely to your plan. Give yourself this week to strengthen these simple actions so you can go on to succeed with further steps. This is important in order to build a healthy foundation. If you feel you have not successfully stuck with your plan, go another week. If you have given yourself a deadline to reach your goals, that's fine, so long as you don't become discouraged along the way. Don't let your rate of progress (or lack of it) become a deterrent for continuing on your path. Your body will always be with you; other plans in your life can be changed!

HERE IS A REVIEW OF YOUR ACTIONS FOR LEVEL IV:

1. Review your positive and motivational points each day.
2. Drink lots of water every day.
3. Substitute fruits or vegetables as snacks or between meals.
4. Do some form of exercise for fifteen minutes each day.
5. Start using a journal or diary to write down your thoughts and feelings.

LEVEL V
Healthy Breakfast

By now you have started to feel—mentally and physically—the changes that are taking place as a result of your simple actions. You should feel a bit of urgency to move to the next level; you should feel ready to do more than the few actions you have taken to this point. That's good. Like a child who feels she has conquered the easy part of a game and wants to get to doing more, or the horse chomping at the bit wanting to break out of the starting gate and run, you should have the desire to go on. Don't you feel different now? Can you see that this is not like any other "diet" you have ever tried? Are you starting to understand why this book is called *Awaken the Diet Within?* You are not ready to break into a full gallop yet, but how about a trot?

It's now time to plan some healthy meals for the week. Not all the meals, just one. Let's start with the most important meal of the day: breakfast. If you're not eating breakfast, or have no set time you can identify as breakfast because your eating is sporadic throughout the day, it's time to make time and a plan for it. Your first meal is important to give your body the nutrition and fuel necessary for the day's activities. You might wake up and not feel like eating breakfast until later, and then you'll be too hungry to eat a moderate meal or too rushed to prepare something healthy. This is not a good place to be, as you will find yourself grabbing anything to satisfy your hunger and will probably consume too much of an unhealthy food. I think this accounts for the majority of office doughnut consumption. If you weren't starving, would you really want to put a blob of fried lard and flour coated with fatty sugar or icing into your body? Leave the oil slicks to the driveway. Taking the time to eat breakfast might be a hurdle you have to get over, but in the end you will see great benefits from planning a healthy first meal.

I didn't realize how important breakfast was until I was well into my weight loss. Only after I found out how many grams of fat were contained in the "healthy" bran muffins I was eating did I start to think about what and when I was actually eating. My appetite was growing during the day as my activity level increased, and therefore I was looking to eat more. I realized the right thing to do was to have a healthy breakfast in preparation for all the activities I would be doing during the day, so I would have the energy and would *not* have the increased appetite. In this way, I would be eating more during the first part of the day, and less at night. Of course you don't want to be consuming more food later in the day, when you're going to be winding down and eventually going to sleep. You don't use much energy when you are sleeping. Food is converted to energy for our body, and if you don't use that energy right away, it gets stored. Stored energy is what we call fat. A great deal of the weight we add comes from eating during the few hours before sleeping. Once I realized this, I was ready for a healthy breakfast and actually started to feel much better during the day.

I recommend choosing a few items you will enjoy. Some of my suggestions can be found at the end of this book. Plan on sticking to egg whites, maybe one egg yolk, a piece of toast, a piece of fruit, and maybe a glass of skim milk. I have a couple of smoothie recipes, although I would recommend having solid food before graduating to smoothies, which may leave you feeling hungry soon after. If you like ham, pick up some low-fat, low-salt ham and have it with your egg whites, along with a sprinkle of low-fat cheese. Add a piece of fruit and you have a healthy start to your day. Oatmeal with fruit is also a great option, or a natural cereal (non–sugar coated) with fruit. If you like coffee or tea, drinking a moderate amount of it in the morning can also jump-start your metabolism and help the calorie-burning process (be careful—like most things in excess, too much coffee or tea can have undesirable effects, making you hungry or jittery).

Keep your meal simple and manageable. Make it something you will enjoy so you don't feel denied, and be sure to plan for the week. Pick up what you need for your breakfast for the entire week. You may be thinking, "Shouldn't I be planning what I eat for lunch and dinner, too?" The answer is yes, but don't change what you've been doing yet. You've already made some substantial changes, believe it or not, and you don't want to overwhelm yourself. It will be a natural progression when you start to feel good enough to stop eating the fast food, the pizzas, and all the other high-calorie foods that you'll notice keep you down and make you feel tired. Don't put your changes into overdrive, only to run out of gas soon after. Eventually you may start to eat less of what you already eat, and that's good. A time will come when it just won't make sense to you to be working out, drinking water, eating healthier foods most of the day, and then ordering a hamburger and fries for dinner. Human beings are creatures of logic, so trust your instincts and let them work to your benefit. Your body is going to love the new way you are caring for it, and it will want more and more of the same.

Continue this week to focus on making a healthy breakfast for yourself, your partner or spouse, and your children if you have them—heck, how about your roommate! We can all stand to get healthier. You may have to endure disgruntled faces in the morning at first, but if you have been slowly changing their lifestyle along with yours, you just may be able to stealth this one in. My daughter loves egg whites and honeydew and cantaloupe in the morning. If I had mentioned it was "healthy" when I started feeding her this way, I might have encountered a fight, but I simply changed what we all were eating. I can't remember being her age and having a good breakfast like that. (Because of my bad habits, she started her first few years learning the same unhealthy bad habits, which led to weight gain. Her weight has leveled off and she looks and feels great since I have changed my lifestyle—that was 1995 and she is thirteen now. As with all teens, her eyes are rolling as I speak of her, so I will stop. Although, like all mothers, I could talk about her or show you pictures all day!

Make your plan for a healthy breakfast for each day of the week. Be proud and happy that you have made the effort and are moving toward your goal. Sit and read your positive and motivating points while you eat, keeping focused on what's good today and what will be better in the future!

HERE IS A REVIEW OF YOUR ACTIONS FOR LEVEL V:

1. Review your positive and motivational points each day.
2. Drink lots of water every day.
3. Substitute fruits or vegetables as snacks or between meals.
4. Do some form of exercise for fifteen minutes each day.
5. Record your thoughts and feelings in a journal.
6. Eat a healthy breakfast each day.

LEVEL VI
More of the Same

In Level VI your goal is to continue with your current actions so as to make them good habits. The longer you continue these simple steps, the easier they will become, and the easier it will be to make more changes. Try adding time to the exercise routine you're doing. Put in at least twenty minutes per day with your walking or the activity you have chosen. Maybe you're ready to try joining a gym and spending twenty minutes each day on the treadmill or another cardio machine: StairMaster, elliptical machine, or stationary bike. Make an extra effort to put exercise at the forefront of your efforts. Your long-term goal is to be able to do forty-five minutes per day. If you stick with only these few actions and increase the time you exercise, you will notice significant changes. If you did nothing else but what you are doing now, I promise you will notice results to be proud of within six months. Think how quickly New Year's Day, or any other holiday, seems to come each year. Plan to continue your resolve until the next holiday. Focus on that short time frame if you feel some difficulty at this time. Don't think about having to do this forever; just focus on the short term. The long term will take care of itself if you are succeeding with your short-term goals. View your actions as something you *get* to do, not *have* to do. Make it enjoyable. It's not that long— you'll be there before you know it.

Again, this level is for continuing to make your actions habits, so you don't need to think twice about doing them. Pay more attention to exercise at this level. You should begin to feel the great benefits of getting your body moving each day!

In addition to the benefits your body is experiencing, let's work on your mind a bit more, too. How about detailing more in your journal, or writing a letter to an old friend you may not have kept in close contact with over the years. Another great thing to do is a random act of kindness for a stranger. You will love how these actions make you feel.

LEVEL VII
One Step Further

You should feel confident about being able to continue and succeed with your efforts at this point. Even if the weight you have lost is not yet substantial, your body will catch up to your habits by dropping weight eventually. Even losing four to five pounds a month after two months equates to eight to ten pounds, and after six months twenty-four to thirty pounds, and after one year sixty pounds! The reality is that once your habits are established, you can begin to challenge yourself in ways that once seemed too much to handle. And this will further accelerate your weight loss beyond what you lost the first month. Challenge yourself to more time or distance with your exercise. Over the next two weeks or so, increase your intensity a bit to work up to thirty minutes. The most important part of exercising is to continue your movements without stopping. You should not be out of breath; if you are you're going too fast and you'll feel overworked. Keep this in mind: Duration is more important than perspiration. Easy exercise, like walking, for at least 30 minutes will be better for you in the long run than running for three minutes as fast as you can. Keeping your heart and breathing rate up will burn calories and help you lose fat. If you can focus on building up the time you put into some form of physical activity, you will feel the benefits almost immediately: more energy, a better attitude, and clearer thinking.

In addition to adding time to your daily exercise, you may now make another change in your diet. I want you to start replacing some of the breads you have for lunch and dinner—any breads, including muffins, pizzas, and rolls. Cookies, cakes, bagels, biscuits, and crackers are all examples of breads you may be eating. I want you to replace these breads with something else. My suggestion is to replace them with a salad, one that has a lot of healthy things like lettuce, vegetables, carrots, strawberries, tomatoes, onions, some Parmesan cheese sprinkles, and low-fat dressing or balsamic vinegar–based dressing. In "Recipes" in Part VII I give you some examples of the great salads I love to make every day. If you don't like salad or can't eat it, find a vegetable or vegetables you do enjoy to replace the breads. Your health pyramid will not be complete without adequate amounts of vegetables, and this is a way to get the necessary quantity in your daily intake without feeling that you're eating bland and boring foods.

Pick up the ingredients you need to have a salad for lunch each day of the week and bring it to the office on Monday. If you need variety without changing your plan, try different dressings. Supermarkets have salad bars that can make a salad an easy item to put together. Do not make the mistake of assuming that anything at the salad bar is a healthy item, though. Avoid mayonnaise-based pasta salads and gelatin molds with whipped cream.

The changes at Level VII will probably take a couple weeks or more to integrate into your lifestyle. Take your time and make sure you are comfortable with these changes before you move on.

HERE IS A REVIEW OF YOUR ACTIONS FOR LEVEL VII :

1. Review your positive and motivational points each day.
2. Drink lots of water every day.
3. Substitute fruits or vegetables as snacks or between meals.
4. Do some form of exercise for at least thirty minutes each day.
5. Record your thoughts and feelings in a journal.
6. Eat a healthy breakfast each day.
7. Replace your lunch and dinner breads with a salad or vegetable.

Take the next two weeks to develop these good habits further. Increasing your exercise and adding roughage (salad and vegetables) to your diet will enhance your weight-loss efforts and bring you to a new level of health.

LEVEL VIII
Getting Stronger

Now that you're getting healthy, your heart and lungs are stronger, your metabolism is operating at a higher level, your energy has increased, your mind is clearer, and you're starting to lose weight, it's time to take your health and fitness to a new level. By now, you probably have been working on your new lifestyle for at least two months, and I'm sure the time has gone quickly, but hopefully not so quickly that you are feeling overwhelmed. If you're not ready for this level, if you are happy continuing with the actions you have already implemented, then do just that for now. Don't fall into a rut but, by the same token, don't leave yourself without some challenge. If you have not built a strong foundation with your current actions and you are still being tested to follow the tasks at hand, by all means continue until you have mastered each level. There is nothing wrong with taking more time to get it right rather than trying to rush, which can result in your becoming frustrated with your progress and giving up. Developing healthy daily habits is more important than just losing weight. The weight loss will be the by-product of a change in lifestyle. But if you are ready, it's time to go further with your exercise program. I'm talking about strengthening your muscles.

An article I recently read at the health club where I exercise explained that weight training burns 500 percent more calories than you would if you were doing only cardiovascular exercise (treadmill, walking, stationary bike). The reason for this is that muscle requires a large number of calories in order to function. The more muscle you have, the more calories you burn. In addition, when muscles are put under stress (exercised), they need to repair, recover, and rebuild themselves—this all burns more calories over time. When you do cardiovascular exercise, you burn calories only while exercising, and for a short while after. However, when you strength-train, your muscles will burn calories all day, increasing your metabolism in the long run. Don't worry that weight training will bulk you up and make you look like a female wrestler. What will really happen is that you will look more toned, burn calories more efficiently, and feel stronger.

Therefore, you need to take actions to begin to strengthen your muscles, above and beyond the exercise you are doing now. Simple, easy-to-follow exercises that you can do in your home are sufficient. You should strive for twenty to forty minutes of strength training three to four times a week. As you begin your strength training, be mindful of rotating exercises for different muscle groups. One day work your arms, shoulders, and back, then work your legs, buttocks, and abdominal muscles the next day. You can purchase resistance rubber bands and three- to ten-pound free weights and develop a routine that will garner great results. In "Resources" you will find my favorite exercise books and tapes.

My preference is to work out at a gym. If you can, join a gym and utilize the machines they have. These machines will allow you better control and more stability in your movements, and the ability to monitor your progress. If you are looking to lose a substantial amount of weight and you fear being in a gym, I suggest starting with the easy at-home exercises. Later, when you gain confidence in your abilities, you can move your exercise program to a gym or purchase additional pieces of at-home equipment. This will keep you from being deterred by an intimidating gym environment or complicated equipment. If you have an all-male or all-female gym in your area, join that one. There's no need to be made up to go exercise, sweating is okay, and it is great building camaraderie with others. My home gym is my best "reward" yet!

Just as in Level VII, these changes will probably take some getting used to. Give yourself at least one month to incorporate strength training into your lifestyle before moving on to Level IX.

HERE IS A REVIEW OF YOUR ACTIONS FOR LEVEL VIII:

1. Review your positive and motivational points each day.
2. Drink lots of water every day.
3. Substitute fruits or vegetables as snacks or between meals.
4. Do some form of exercise for at least thirty minutes each day, adding muscle strengthening—rotating body parts every day, i.e., doing legs one day, arms the next.
5. Record your thoughts and feelings in a journal.
6. Eat a healthy breakfast each day.
7. Replace your lunch and dinner breads with a salad or vegetable.

LEVEL IX
Going the Extra Mile

By now you are following the basic eating plan, which consists of making a few changes from your previous menu. Your daily schedule includes exercising, which has given you more energy, more confidence, and a better overall feeling of health. No matter how much weight you have lost, your daily routine should be sound at this point. Your fitness level in the weeks to come will become very noticeable to you and others. I remember how, a few weeks after beginning an exercise program—I was doing aerobics at the time—my energy level and attitude had grown exponentially from the time I started. If you don't already feel this way, you will. It's just a matter of time.

If you are now ready to go a step farther in your commitment to health and fitness, I suggest you join a gym if you have not already done so. If that is not an option for you, make an investment in a good piece of at-home exercise equipment. I recommend equipment that exercises your muscles, as opposed to buying a treadmill, stationary bike, or other cardio items, unless you have the room and the money to buy both. The alternative is to buy a treadmill (or another cardio machine) and join a gym to use the muscle-strengthening machines. This way you don't miss a beat when your schedule may not permit going to the gym every day, and you can always take the time to walk on your treadmill at home. Alternate days you use the strengthening machines with the days you do only cardio. But be sure you spend five minutes doing cardio to warm up on the days you do muscle strengthening. The point of these actions is to keep your focus on your fitness, not just on losing weight.

Looking at the plan to this point, it is apparent that exercise carries as much if not more "weight" than a complete and detailed eating plan when it comes to losing weight and getting fit. As we've already noted, our lives are very sedentary compared to decades ago, when machines were not as prevalent and we had to do more physical activity to complete a regular job or task. Exercise puts us back at that level of activity and more. Sticking to daily exercise will definitely accelerate your weight loss, although in order to reach an optimum level of health your diet will need to be a healthy one as well.

The next step to completing your health pyramid should be a well-defined eating plan. Is this step necessary for losing weight? Actually, no. The changes you have already made will lead to weight loss. Is it necessary to achieve a fit and healthy body and maintain it for life? Yes! This level is where most diet plans begin. Starting at this point overwhelms us by the changes that are demanded, thereby causing us to fail at our efforts. I read a diet book recently in which the author wanted the reader to pick a date to start her diet and circle it on the calendar. Then the night before the start date the reader was to take a few moments to think of the new life she would begin in the morning. Then, in the morning, everything changed for this person. Or at least that is what the author intended. One day the reader was eating burgers, fries, and soft drinks, and the next she was expected to be the epitome of healthy eating, staying under 1,300 calories a day.

Aren't you thankful now that you have gotten many weeks of setting healthy habits ingrained in you? Don't you think that the past weeks have solidified your resolve and that you will now be able to make another change more easily? I hope so. I believe people should not attempt this level until after a number of weeks of working up to it. Your eating schedule should now consist of planned meals for the week that include fruits and proteins (e.g., eggs) for breakfast; salads, meats, and a small amount of bread or carbohydrates for lunch; vegetables, meats, or fish, and a small amount of carbohydrates (e.g., baked potato) for dinner. This can be beneficial when it comes to saving time and keeping it simple. You can follow the menu I have laid out for you or you can choose from the recipes in Part VII. You do not have to stick to them solely or forever, but do use them for the next few weeks, until you are more clearly aware of what healthy food looks, tastes, and smells like. My philosophy is to keep things simple and easy, but this level is for you who choose to get the A+ in health and fitness. You can remain forever at the previous level, achieve a B, and find that you feel good, look good, are confident with yourself, and can do all the things you once felt were impossible.

You can also slack off and revert to some of your old habits and get a C, or you can slowly allow all of your old vices to take charge of you again and get a D. Worse still would be never even to attempt Level I and fail with an F. *You will never know what you are capable of until you try. If you fail to try, you will only know what you are not capable of.*

Today, I feel as though I live solidly on Level IX with an A- on most days and a B on others. My day starts with a breakfast of egg whites and some fruit (often cantaloupe), then I go to the gym in the morning, where I alternate between using the strengthening machines and cardio one day, and doing only the cardio machines (elliptical machine or treadmill) the next. For lunch I eat a big salad with many different types of vegetables and a light dressing, and during the afternoon I will snack on an apple and sometimes eat some chicken breast with some light sauce or a hard-boiled egg, white only (these are proteins or fruits). For dinner I will eat a piece of chicken, lean meat, or fish with some steamed asparagus or another vegetable, and at night when I'm working on my computer I may have some no-butter, no-salt popcorn. Throughout the entire day I have my water bottle within reach. If you have seen me you know I do not have a supermodel body, and some would say that I could still lose ten pounds—that may be a result of the occasional gourmet coffees and chocolate-chip cookies. But I am very healthy and happy, I have a high energy level, and I am very active.

You too can live on this level and be proud of your health and fitness. It is only after you have taken the time to make small changes and developed some simple, healthy habits that you should attempt Level IX. It is at this level that you can graduate to extended time in the health club, purchasing your own equipment, following a more regimented eating plan or joining a diet group, and paying more attention to your health. The actions at this level are the ones that will get you to your ideal weight over time and quite possibly to the body of your dreams. Not everyone has the time, the genes, and the ability to have the "perfect" body (however we define such a body). And certainly if you look at the time frame here, you are only at your third month of this plan, and it's probably not realistic for most of you to think that you are close to your weight-loss goals, and it may not be fair to talk about achieving the body of your dreams. But these are, in fact, the actions that will give you total health and fitness. Keeping consistent with your plan and keeping your diet simple will get you more than 80 percent of the way there. It is only after this point that you can tailor your diet and your exercise to address specifically the final ten to twenty pounds of your weight-loss goal. I get a lot of E-mail from women wanting to lose that last ten pounds—so do I! To do so requires going farther than Level IX; it takes strict commitment and no straying (gourmet coffee and cookies would be banned for me). And that is not for me. It may be what you want, but decide that after you reach total compliance with this level. Get at or close to your goal weight and stay there for a few months before you decide if you need to lose more. My guess is that you will be so happy you won't have a complaint in the world. I promise you that if you never go past this level in your life you will still experience successful weight loss. It just takes persistence, and therefore time.

TIME

You're probably reading this book all the way through and not taking action yet, and that's okay. It's sort of like fortune-telling: You will know what is going to happen to you next. You can go back and begin taking steps after you finish reading. But keep in mind that this book is a guideline. The steps to get started should not change, although the time frame to complete a level and move on to the next can fluctuate. This is why I have categorized them as levels as opposed to specific lengths of time. You can complete a level with consistency, look back each week, and evaluate your efforts. You decide if it is time to move on. View each level as a block of time in which to make the effort to complete each small endeavor. Even if you don't proceed to the next level, be sure that you evaluate your actions on a week-to-week basis. If it takes you three months to get to Level V, that's great! It means that you have stuck to your plan and made progress. Think of this as something that is happening in your life without your paying much attention. It sounds ironic, but if you are overweight by sixty-five pounds or more, you probably have not paid a lot of constructive attention to exercise and eating healthfully. You may feel that all you have done is think about weight, but if your approach has been wrong, all you have really done is waste time. If you think that simply putting more time and attention into your health and diet plan will make you lose weight more quickly, you may be mistaken. This will just make you more frustrated because you won't see the changes you want relative to the amount of time you are putting in— weight loss takes time! Do the simple, easy actions to start, and then work your way up to a higher level of exercise and weight training, and then proceed to meal planning and calorie counting.

The simple, commonsense approach will be the most successful. Focus less on the amount of time that it takes to reach your goals, and more on the simple, healthy actions that you are doing to improve the overall quality of your life. It took me fifteen months to lose my 130 pounds. If you are getting on the scale more than once a week, you are trying to defy nature's time frame. Be patient; know that by staying firmly on the path of Self-Improvement through Self-Motivation, you will realize your dreams in due time.

Remember, this level is for those who desire an optimal level of physical fitness. There are even more levels if your goals include running a marathon, becoming a fitness model, or competing in a fitness contest. The question is how far do you want to go? Keep in mind that those with the perfectly sculpted bodies are usually those whose job or career depends on it. And at what level do you think these people are living when it comes to diet and exercise? Not a level I am interested in. Stick with these basic actions and you will feel triumphant about the level of mental and physical health you will achieve!

HERE IS A REVIEW OF YOUR ACTIONS FOR LEVEL IX:

1. Review your positive and motivational points each day.
2. Start your day with a healthy breakfast.
3. Drink lots of water.
4. Eat plenty of fruits, vegetables, and salads during meals and as snacks.
5. Record your thoughts and feelings in a journal.
6. Join a gym and/or purchase home exercise equipment.
7. Exercise five or six days a week, alternating days of strength training and cardiovascular workouts.
8. Follow my meal and eating plan, or your own version, using my recipes. You will find this plan at the end of the book with the grocery list and recipes.

The Ten Dos and Don'ts of Healthy Living

Let's get the bad out of the way first. *The don'ts:*

1. Don't diet. The first three letters in "diet" should tell you it's not good.

2. Don't go too fast. Change takes time; be patient.

3. Don't get overwhelmed. Forget about the weight and think about the actions.

4. Don't be hard on yourself. We learn from mistakes and our life experiences.

5. Don't be negative. Use negative emotions to get going toward being positive.

6. Don't cheat. There are no shortcuts to health but many fast roads to death.

7. Don't count. Counting calories will make you crazy and takes too much time.

8. Don't waste time. You have a finite amount of time on earth—get busy now!

9. Don't put junk in. Remember garbage in equals garbage out—avoid junk food.

10. Don't forget! Remember who you are and what you desire to be—every day.

Now for the good stuff. *The dos:*

1. **Do the right thing.** The right thing is whatever makes you healthier in any way.

2. **Do drink lots of water.** Our bodies are two-thirds water— you figure it out!

3. **Do eat healthfully.** Eat a balance of fruits, veggies, meats and fish, and some breads and carbohydrates every day.

4. **Do exercise.** Our bodies were made to move, so move it!

5. **Do think positive.** Increasing your energy starts with increasing your positive thoughts.

6. **Do envision a picture.** Know what your life as a more fit and healthy person will look like.

7. **Do keep it simple.** Just take one step at a time, and build on each step.

8. **Do the basics.** Keep the big picture in mind; everything you do should support it.

9. **Do have weekly goals.** Accomplishing things one week at a time will make it easier.

10. **Do it now!** This is not a dress rehearsal—this is the real thing—so make it right!

PART V

———

———

Maintaining the
New You

Maintaining health requires us to have a handle on all areas of our life, regardless of where we are in our fitness level. There are many hurdles that may come our way—temptations that are put before us, or changes and added stresses to our life—that can upset our daily routine. You need to have some safety nets in place so that if and when things do change, you are prepared. Let's go over ways to stay on track when facing some common challenges.

Learning the Life of Health

I am often sent messages from people who tell me that they "lost the weight a year or two ago and had kept it off for about six months, only to gain it all back again and more." They explain how something changed in their life and now they are back to being sixty pounds overweight. We have a name for this: yo-yo dieting. The last thing anyone who has been overweight wants to do is put the weight back on after losing it. Why is it that after we have wanted to lose weight for so long and have taken the necessary steps to do so, we gain the weight back? Often it is because we revert back to our old ways and habits, the very same lifestyle that got us overweight in the first place. If you stop to think about this logically for a moment, it makes perfect sense. We thought our old ways were "normal" and that we were just "fat." Once we lost the weight, we felt we were "cured" and could then be "normal" again. I think I have successfully stressed in this book that a healthy lifestyle is what must now be considered normal and adhered to for life. Anything other than that will leave you continually living on the yo-yo-dieting cycle.

One of the most common reasons for gaining weight back after losing it is lack of a permanent lifestyle change. We go on a diet and temporarily change to accommodate the program, but we fail to learn how to live a healthy life. When our goal weight is reached and we have crossed the "finish line," we can now go off the diet and go back to living "normally" again. We all know where that leads—back to where we came from. I'm sure you can see the problem: If you go *on* a diet, at some point you will go *off* the diet. Once you go "off" of it you can't continue to eat as though you are still on it. The successful approach consists of changing your whole lifestyle to one of health and fitness.

In order to maintain your weight loss and continue progressing toward your desired weight, you must learn to enjoy a healthy lifestyle and remember the reasons why you wanted to be healthy in the first place (look at your motivation list—refer to it often). Do these reasons still apply to you today? Do you need to add to them or revise them to suit your place in life today? This is an action you can do now to help you stay focused on all the positive reasons for maintaining a healthy lifestyle. Find someone to share the same goals and activities with you, someone with whom you can exercise each day so you can encourage each other. Being on the elliptical machine for forty-five minutes at my health club is much easier with a friend next to me who is doing the same. When your attention is taken away from the effort of completing forty-five minutes, you will find it not only easier but also more enjoyable with a workout partner. You can make it a game to see who goes farther if you're both using a treadmill. Or challenge each other to continue forty-five minutes without stopping. Either way, a partner makes exercise more enjoyable, and it's easier to stay committed to a lifestyle of health with one. If I am exercising alone, I always bring a novel to read. I can effortlessly stay on the machine for an hour and almost hate that it's over and I have to close my beloved book. With young children in the house, this hour is my solitude and private time. Enjoy it—don't make it a chore.

A second, lesser-known reason why we often gain the weight back and become unhealthy again is that we no longer have a goal or goals that are challenging us to succeed. If we have succeeded with our weight loss, or are near enough that we don't have the same motivation we had when we started, it's easier to get complacent. After all, we feel we're in control now that we've lost some weight, so we can handle a day off. After repeating these "lazy" days several times, we then begin to gain an unnoticeable amount of weight, which gives us no alert to get back on track.

Another reason we do this to ourselves, even subconsciously, is to provide a new challenge, to make things difficult and to provide us with a goal again, and a renewed motivation to get fit. You can be so used to living overweight and obsessing about your weight that you may not know what to do as you get closer to getting fit. After all, if you feel you have gotten what you set out to get, where does the motivation come from to stay fit? You don't have a challenge to lose weight if you've already lost it, right? Subconsciously, you may be acting to self-destruct in order to revert to a lifestyle with which you are more familiar. You need to be ready when that time comes so you have your motivation (goals) in place to stay fit. After all, we don't want to work hard to arrive at the top of the mountain, merely glance at the view, and immediately go back down. Let's stay at the top and continue to enjoy the view: the healthy and fit lifestyle.

Keeping Motivated to Stay Fit

After losing the weight, we tend to believe that we can eat all the junk food we want today because we won't gain all the weight back in one day. After all, we're pretty fit now, and one day of unhealthy eating won't change things noticeably. Well, one day this week becomes two days next week, and so on, until we suddenly begin to notice extra weight—maybe twenty pounds or more. Remember, you never set out to become obese in the first place; it happened one bite at a time, and if you do not stay on the defensive, it will steal its way back on again.

Once you are at or near your goal, your motivation and commitment to fitness and health should come from doing the things you enjoy now that you're fit. You should do the things you once longed to become capable of doing—and being—with more energy and a better shape. You must do the things that will reinforce your healthy lifestyle. It is important to define why you want to have better health, increased energy, and a slimmer body so that there is no doubt in your mind that you won't return to your old way of life. In this way you will be able to handle the most common bump in the road when it comes to keeping fit, and that is keeping motivated.

There are a couple of things, for example, that keep me motivated to stay fit: I enjoy having the energy to do activities with my kids. I bought them a trampoline for their birthdays (which are close together), and I was able to jump on it with them. Also, my husband is very fit and in shape, and that increases my desire to be fit so we can enjoy the same things together: riding bikes, skiing, or just taking a walk.

I dreamed of being in a beauty pageant as a teen. What woman doesn't watch Miss America and dream it could be her? After losing weight, my husband encouraged me to enter the Mrs. Missouri pageant. And I won! After being awarded the title, I had to compete nationally for the Mrs. USA crown. Just the thought of this kept me motivated to be as fit as possible, in order to look as good as I could in comparison to the other women. I didn't win the Mrs. USA title, but I can tell you this: It felt great to be in a swimsuit on that stage at the Rio Hotel in Las Vegas and know that I was fit and healthy. Not to mention the fact that a few years earlier I had weighed 290 pounds! Talk about a dream come true. Even without the crown and bouquet of roses I came away a winner.

These are just a few examples of how I've kept motivated and stayed on track. Continue to set new goals and plans for yourself. Think about what you want to do in life and how much more you can improve. After all, as we age there is always something about our health we can improve upon.

Not Letting Your Emotions Rule Your Appetite

One of the most difficult things we confront when it comes to managing our weight is avoiding eating for emotional reasons. When you find yourself angry or depressed, or happy and excited, keep mindful of why you are reaching for food. We all have a tendency to eat when certain emotions come over us: If we are happy and we're celebrating the holidays with family, it's time to sit down and eat and be joyous. If we have had bad news—a relative is dying, for instance—we may reach for something to eat to seek solace in food. The point is to be very careful not to let your emotions control your appetite. You didn't suddenly become hungry; your state of mind just changed. I'm sure you know someone who has a cigarette when they are stressed out, or people may appear to be in a good mood while they're smoking. For many, cigarettes seem to offer a diversion from pains and pleasures. The same holds true for many of us who have had extra weight. We eat to change the way we feel, or to celebrate the way we feel. Food becomes a constant in the sea of emotions that is our life, and we come to rely on food when things are really bad or really good. There were more times than I care to remember when eating was the center of my emotions—I ate to feel better when I was down, and to feel good about being up (on the days I was happy). And my anger was also directly connected to food. Once I realized *why* I was eating I became more in control of the situation and was able to break this habit. Moderation needs to guide your actions. Try to stop and think about your pending action and ask yourself, "Will this cupcake really improve my mood and the problem at hand, or will it just make matters worse?" The answer will be the latter, so drop the cupcake!

One of the easiest ways I have found to handle stress and difficult emotions (like anger or apathy) is to get some exercise (again?). Yes, if my day has been an example of Murphy's Law—anything that can go wrong will go wrong—I find that going to the health club and spending time on my machine of choice (elliptical) will relieve my stress and allow me to think more clearly. How about taking a kickboxing class to get out some aggression or buying a pair of boxing gloves for the occasion? If you're depressed, turn your depression into anger and use that energy to get up and get moving. Even if it's just to take a walk, walk at a fast pace. Or—my favorite—tickle your kids! Nothing I have ever eaten can bring a smile to my heart as quickly as a child's laughter.

A more luxurious suggestion, which may be a little more appealing to you, is a massage. A massage is a great way to handle a stressful day. If this is not practical or affordable, try taking a hot bath. A bath will relieve tension and stress too. Other possibilities are a yoga class, meditation, or even prayer. On the other side of the emotion coin, if you're feeling good about your day or any of your successes, do something healthy and positive. This would be considered a reward—see "Rewards" at the end of Part III for details. If you find yourself stuck in a rut and you just can't get out of it, then it is time to deploy this defense: Volunteer somewhere. Find a charity or service that will benefit from your time, treasure, or talent and give yourself to it. Nothing in the world will make you feel as wonderful as giving to others. It is the best way I know to gain a more balanced perspective on your life and what may seem at the moment to be the weight of the world on your shoulders. Look around your world—there are others who need your help so much more than you need that cupcake. Giving to them will return much more to you in the long run. Anything you can do to keep your emotions (good or bad) detached from food will help you act in a healthy way.

Satisfying the Occasional Sweet Tooth

I am often asked how to deal with the unhealthy foods that are difficult to give up, most commonly sweets. Women often tell me they know they should not eat something, yet they can't give it up and don't know what to do. My recommendation is to find an alternative if possible that cuts down the quantity of their vice substantially. In other words, if you like to have chocolate and don't want to give it up completely, find a source of chocolate that will satisfy your urge while limiting the calories. One good example is carrying two or three Hershey's Kisses with you and making a point to limit yourself to those for the entire day. (I keep them in the freezer and can savor one for up to twenty minutes as it slowly melts in my mouth.) Remember, it is the taste you are craving, not the quantity. Ultimately, if you can give up the sweets completely, you will feel more in control. If you know you are consuming too much of anything unhealthy, take steps to wean yourself off the item. Remember not to overwhelm yourself with change. I will give you this little secret about consuming sweets that you may not know: If you are putting in thirty to forty-five minutes per day of exercise and you are consistent with your daily eating plan, you are not going to ruin your fitness level with an occasional treat. Here is another bonus: If you have to fill that occasional urge for a sweet, try to satisfy your sweet tooth just before you exercise. In this way you will be "burning off" these calories before they have a chance to do harm.

When you're in control, practicing good, healthy habits, you can pick up a chocolate knowing it doesn't control *you*. This is the attitude you will have now that you are living a healthy lifestyle.

Dealing with Age

Other obstacles we face when trying to maintain our progress or fitness level are the changes that occur in our bodies as we age. We may know what it's like to be ten pounds lighter, but not one of us knows what it's like to be ten years older. From the experience of others and studies comparing the systems and functions of a twenty-year-old and a forty-year-old, we can better prepare ourselves for what's ahead.

The sooner you start on your healthy lifestyle, the easier it will be to maintain your fitness level as you age. It's easier to lose weight if you are in your twenties than if you are forty or older. But please don't be discouraged if you're older than forty, because you will have greater mental strength than your younger counterpart. (Okay, I can't prove that, but at forty it makes me feel a lot better to say it!)

Regardless of what age you are today, the longer you wait to take control of your fitness level, the more difficult it becomes. This certainly isn't a pep talk, but there is one point I'd like to make: You'll never know how much easier it would have been had you taken action ten years ago, so you don't want to wonder ten years from now what it would have been like if only you had taken action now. As we age, our metabolism slows down and it takes a bit more effort to get going in the morning—to get our heart pumping, our muscles warmed up, and our minds sharp. I am told that if we keep our calorie intake the same and don't change our daily activity level, we will gain an average of two to three pounds per year after the age of thirty-five. This is an average, but if you take that number and multiply it by fifteen years, you've got thirty or more pounds with you.

Taking action to get fit and stay fit every day is the surest way to deal with the added challenge of age. There are all kinds of companies selling us products to deal with our slowing metabolism, the most obvious and well-known result of aging. The healthiest way to boost your metabolism is to exercise. It's a natural effect of getting your body moving every day. If you feel old and are trying to get started on losing weight, don't despair. You will feel like you are turning back the clock as you continue to eat right and exercise. Nature's true fountain of youth will be at work for you. If you have succeeded in realizing your fitness goals, remember that your body will slow down as you age and you may want to increase your exercise level and/or cut some of the calories you're taking in. It's best to be aware of the changes you will go through. If you are older and are struggling to make progress, keep consistent with your actions—be persistent. You may need a little more time to get fit. But, more important, you should feel the benefits of exercise and healthy eating in no time. Your body is probably more sensitive than that of a twenty-year-old.

Another problem to combat as we age is our loss of flexibility. Taking a yoga class or stretching on a daily basis could be the answer. These exercises have more positive benefits than I can list. Stretching alone allows the muscles to get blood and therefore warm up, making it easier for you to get moving and be productive. The amount of flexibility we lose over the years can be made up with regular stretching. Pilates is a very popular form of exercise; its main goal is to stretch the muscles during the workout. I would suggest that you take up a stretching program no matter what your age, but especially if you're over forty. Doing yoga and kickboxing is a plan I implemented the year I turned forty—so far so good. My flexibility is improving and I am learning to calm down at least during class (I am fairly hyper by nature and never relax totally). Good health and fitness can be achieved much faster with better flexibility from stretching. The added bonus of incorporating these into your regimen is that they are very relaxing and soothing to the mind, body, and soul. Things that you may have had difficulty doing before may seem a little easier and possibly more enjoyable. Try yoga, stretching, or Pilates after you have made some progress with your healthy lifestyle changes and built a foundation of basic actions for good health. You won't have any regrets.

Supplements

What would a book about losing weight and getting fit be without mentioning one or more of the millions of diet supplements that are on the market today? While I am a firm believer in keeping things simple and doing the basic things every day to get healthy and keep healthy, I do think supplements have their place. I have tried many diet supplements, stuck with only a few, and found results in even fewer. There is definitely something about taking supplements that we don't like. I've yet to hear someone tell me they've "been taking XYZ supplement for the last year with great success." I'm not referring to a daily vitamin or any nutritional supplement taken to help maintain health or help prevent sickness. I am referring to the supplements we buy with the expectation of rapidly seeing or feeling dramatic weight loss with little to no effort. In my experience, whatever results they offer are usually short-lived.

There are many misconceptions about diet supplements, the most common of which is that we can take something to "burn the fat" and magically take off the weight. Every day I see or hear of a pill or liquid supplement that claims to take off the weight with little or no effort on my part. The advertisements imply that we can eat double cheeseburgers and still lose the sixty pounds. They tout their testimonials about how "easy it was" and how "the pounds just melted away." If you have ever tried one of these supplements you know that, alone, these products don't work—period. Many of these diet supplements contain caffeine and other stimulants, which can cause negative side effects. And some diet supplements can be harmful; we've all become aware of some products that have been taken off the market because of their dangerous side effects. In any case, there is always the fine print that explains that the supplement works only when combined with a healthy eating plan and moderate exercise.

Let's take a commonsense approach. When you reach your weight-loss goal or are close to it, you can try a supplement or two to help you with the last twenty pounds, or to help sculpt your body. These products may make a difference for someone who is exercising hard six days a week and has been for two or three years, but you will probably be discouraged if you're just getting started and have sixty-five or more pounds to lose. I believe most of these diet supplements work best (if at all) for people who are already living at Level VIII—those who want to sculpt their body (lose that last five pounds), want to add muscle, or both. I know I'm not at this point and don't care to be unless I decide to try for the supermodel career and make fitness a full-time job. If you have a unique situation regarding your health, you may want to consult a naturopath or other health-care provider who specializes in herbal and vitamin supplements. Many of the ingredients added to supplements today can make them downright unhealthy. Remember, your journey is one on which you're seeking better health, so do nothing to contradict that.

There are a couple of supplements I would feel comfortable recommending to you, based on the limited amount of knowledge I have regarding the subject. Again, consult your health-care provider before taking any supplements. I mention these based on the positive results I have had using them.

One supplement I used with some good results over time is chitosan. Chitosan is made from shellfish fiber and naturally binds to some of the fat in the food you eat and eliminates it. Chitosan is by no means a fat eraser. You cannot eat an entire key lime pie with your chitosan and still expect to come out on top. However, if you know you are going out and may indulge in something containing more fat than you would usually eat, you can use chitosan. Studies have shown that one gram of chitosan can bind to about four times its weight— four grams of fat. If you have an allergy to shellfish, then this is not for you as it will cause an allergic reaction. If you decide to use it, remember that it is not a license to overeat. And chitosan should not be taken on a daily basis. If you take it before a high-fat meal, you will be left with much of the fat you consumed; it eliminates only some of it. There are many different brands of chitosan and different formulations.

Another supplement, human growth hormone, or HGH, as it's known, seems to offer great promise and hope when it comes to helping to improve our health and helping our fitness efforts. HGH may very well serve the intended purpose of a "supplement": to make up for a deficiency. Human growth hormone exists naturally in our bodies in larger quantities during our growth years, and the levels of HGH in our body decrease substantially after the age of thirty. An HGH supplement can help maintain the body's hormonal balances, which helps it function more efficiently. There are many informative sources of literature on HGH on the Internet, in bookstores, and in health-food stores. I would suggest reading some material and consulting your doctor before deciding if HGH is right for you. (Beware: You just may know more than your doctor when you're done!) I especially like that nowhere in the literature have I read that, while taking HGH, I can "eat all I want and not exercise and still feel great." I still have to do all of the healthy things I can; it just may be helping me do them a bit better.

I strongly recommend a daily multimineral multivitamin supplement to assist your body as it starts to change and requires better nutrition. In addition, it will help counteract all the toxins we breathe and the additives we ingest through foods and beverages over the years. By taking vitamins you will be giving yourself some added health assurance. For the long term, I believe in a daily supplement as maintenance for keeping healthy. How will you ever know if it's doing any good? I suppose you could wait until you're sixty-five and then second-guess yourself about whether things might be different if you had taken daily supplements. With that said, my seventy-year-old father has always taken several vitamins, nutritional supplements, and herbs, including some we have mercilessly teased him for, like bee pollen, alfalfa, and comfrey root. He must know something the rest of us don't because he still plays squash every day, skis with his grandchildren, is working in a very high pressure career, and is at the top of his game. Please pass the comfrey!

As you begin increasing your exercise routine, you put more demands on your body, and therefore a vitamin or nutritional supplement is not a bad idea to support your body's extra needs.

Another emerging supplement today is soy. The benefits of soy are numerous. I have begun adding soy protein to my smoothies. Whether we like it or not, we age. Incorporating healthy items, such as soy, into our diet just may make the effects of the aging process less problematic.

Providing Yourself with New Challenges

The best way to help yourself grow healthier—physically, mentally, spiritually, and even financially—is always to provide yourself with new challenges. Long-term goals should be broad, and you should aim high. Short-term goals we reach almost immediately. By coming up with new challenges that are interesting, motivating, and allow us to grow, we can keep our lives from becoming mundane—and we may never again know the bad habits we once had. The journey that you are embarking on is never-ending; you can and always should be improving, so keep it fun and interesting.

Examples involving exercise are easy to come up with. For example, training to do a 5K run to support a charity is a short-term goal that will help satisfy a long-term one (getting or keeping fit). Or how about entering a pageant?

Another example would be to read a book about a subject of interest. If you want to be able to travel as you become more fit and have more energy, you could read up on the places you want to go. This will help reinforce your goals and your motivation, and support mental health.

Challenge yourself to be more productive at work and try to complete a new goal for the week. Take up a new hobby. Maybe it is time to learn how to play a musical instrument, or become better at the one you play. If art is of interest to you, spend time learning how to paint with oils and create something beautiful for your home. Enroll in a class on a subject of interest at a local community college. That bit of knowledge you gain may give you more ability at your job or with a new hobby or talent. Take a spiritual journey, a retreat to a quiet place. There are many things I'm sure you would like to do that will empower you and give you the strength to continue on your path of self-improvement—a journey of financial, physical, mental, and spiritual health.

I have developed a few fun methods for keeping new challenges fresh. I call the first one Rewards Bingo. To play this, all you need to do is get some three-by-five cards and write the letters B-I-N-G-O on them. Now decide on five weekly goals you want to achieve; these can be as simple as drinking your designated amount of water each day, doing exercise, feeling positive. Each time you successfully realize a goal, you get a letter. At the end of the week, if you have BINGO, shout it out, jump up and down. Be excited. You won! As the Bingo winner, you can give yourself a prize, a reward of your choice.

Another idea about keeping challenges fresh came to me when potty-training my son. His day-care teacher used to use "tinkle stickers" to reward the kids each time they used the potty. She then took it one step farther and had tissue "targets" that she placed in the water for the boys, getting them trained to "hit the target" rather than being messy. Each day my son would come home as proud as the most decorated military hero displaying the array of colorful stickers that were strewn about his T-shirt. I created my own sticker system. I made a collage out of cut-up pictures from magazines showing the clothes I wanted to wear, the body I wanted to have. I pasted large letters that spelled positive affirmation words all over it, along with photos of my children. Each time I stayed positive—said affirmations to myself rather than making an unhealthy choice—I got another sticker. When the month was over, if my collage was completed, it was like cashing in the old Green Stamps. I used the collages to help make my rewards plan tangible and visible. Rather than allowing the measure on the scale to be my indicator of success, I let my collection of stickers serve as a visible indicator of my progress as well. I would reward myself with things like a trip to the movies or a new exercise outfit. I still utilize rewards today to help me meet new challenges.

Julia's Rules for Staying Positive

1. ALWAYS KEEP THE BIG PICTURE IN MIND

It is very easy to get consumed with all the little things going on in our lives and we forget about the "big picture." I'm sure you've heard the two rules "Don't sweat the small stuff" and "It's all small stuff." We all have things to take care of, like getting groceries, picking up gifts, shopping for school clothes, and so on, that can keep our focus off of the big picture of our life. In the hustle and bustle each day, don't forget things like the Golden Rule. In times of trouble and despair, how we treat others will certainly go farther than any one accomplishment we could be working so hard for.

2. SET MEANINGFUL STANDARDS AND VALUES FOR SUCCESS

Setting standards that are meaningful to you will let you know at what level you wish to live your life, and where you can grow from there. For instance, set standards for how much time you want to devote each day to such things as exercise, reading, prayer, reviewing goals. You can order these standards on which of these you value most in your life. That way you have set priorities regarding which aspect is most important to you, and which needs more attention. In this way you will establish a strong foundation for success, and you will stay focused on a healthy path.

Having balance comes from having set standards that you act on each day to keep each area of your life strong. We may spend more time doing something that supports our basic needs, like working at a job to make money to eat, even though it may not come first on our list of what is most important in our life. In other words, don't leave out what is important just because it may not take much time to do, like not taking the time to eat something healthy: Although it may not hurt today, repeatedly, over the course of weeks, lacking a healthy meal will eventually cause you to gain extra weight and have poorer health. Don't leave anything behind when it comes to growing. Grow stronger and healthier in every way—mentally, spiritually, physically, financially, and socially.

3. STAY FOCUSED ON WHERE YOU'RE GOING, NOT WHERE YOU'VE BEEN

Many times readers tell me they can't get over having done this, that, or the other. They tell me their life story and how difficult things were for several reasons, and it has all added up to being 100 pounds overweight. It's not always easy to look ahead and forget about what has happened in the past, but it's a step well worth taking. Sometimes I think we must do an about-face. Everything that has happened *to* us keeps us mesmerized on past events, forgetting to take action now to make our future better. In the movie *IQ*, one of Einstein's friends makes the argument that there is no present or future because each future moment becomes a present one, which immediately becomes a past moment. Therefore there is no present or future, but only a past. (Either way, it's confusing!) It makes me think that we must act now because those future moments keep coming and going with no regard for how little or much we're paying attention. Plan for the future so you can look forward to what's to come!

4. SURROUND YOURSELF WITH THE POSITIVE

Turn on any television, open any newspaper, listen to any radio, and there are plenty of stories about negative things going on in our world. It's very easy to be influenced by seeing and hearing all kinds of stories that may cause anger, resentment, sadness, fear, and sympathy. If you allow these emotions to overcome you, it is quite easy to resort to overeating, to seemingly soothe the pain of life. Reject that line of thinking. Limit the amount of time you spend watching the news on TV or listening to the news on the radio. The newspaper can be a more digestible medium, as you can pick and choose what information you wish to consume. But sticking with stories and information that will improve your mood and/or your motivation will be healthier in the long run. For every negative story there are many more positive ones. Even the most devastating tragedies spawn quietly inspirational stories of survival and heroism, but the media tend to focus on the sensational ones, the more horrific ones. Seek out the good word; it is always there if you look hard enough.

Television can be a great source of entertainment that provides us with laughter, yet all the bad news delivered can bring out unhappy emotions. There are plenty of positive stories out there, they just aren't as easy to get at with a remote control. You can find stories about people doing great things, overcoming the odds, succeeding where success was totally unexpected. These are the types of positive influences we want to fill our minds, hearts, and spirits with. This is what will lift our motivational spirits and not oppress them. I would recommend limiting the amount of time watching TV. Not only does it take away from your time to "do," it may also dampen your mood.

Many consider television another item that is making a substantial contribution to the extra weight. I'd be willing to bet that the majority of those seeking to lose weight could reach their goal in less than six months if they exercised instead of watching TV. If you watch TV, try to make it something uplifting. I love to watch *The Shawshank Redemption* or *The Green Mile* if I want a deep message about the spirit of mankind, or *The Birdcage, The Big Lebowski,* or *Planes, Trains & Automobiles* if I want to laugh. Movies can be a great escape—just make sure you do not have butter on your air-popped popcorn!

Make a game of it to see if you can go a week without watching TV. If you try it, be sure to have something ready to replace TV—reading, walking, listening to music (and walking!).

While it may be easy to turn off the TV or radio, or skip a story in the newspaper, the same may not be true for the not-so-positive people in your environment. Try avoiding negative conversation, or what may not be positive or constructive communication. Doing something or saying something nice for or to someone will go a lot farther to improve your own attitude, productivity, and respect for others than saying or doing the opposite. I sometimes find that having a little music in the background while I'm working can put a little pep in my fingers on the keyboard. If you can, use music to keep the "rhythm" of your positive attitude during parts of your day. And be sure to find ways to exert *your* positive influence on those around you.

5. DEVELOP A DAILY ROUTINE TO KEEP YOU ON YOUR PATH

One thing that will be most helpful in your weight-loss efforts, and in achieving any goal, is developing a routine, a routine that consists of always planning the night before what you want to get done tomorrow and when. Get up each day at approximately the same time with the same healthy actions to start the day, maybe some light stretching and reading for fifteen minutes. Get to sleep at approximately the same time each night. I think it's true for most of us that if we aren't sleeping regularly—going to sleep at the same time each night—we're not getting the most out of our potential the next day. I know I don't feel as sharp if my sleep hours are altered from my regular routine.

This doesn't mean you should get in a rut, but you do need to get into the habit of taking actions that are consistent with your goal. If you stick to doing a few simple things every day—drink plenty of water, get some exercise, take steps to be productive—then you can build on your routine to accomplish more. I never really thought that getting things done each day would help realize my dreams; it was only with hindsight that I appreciated the importance of continually moving forward. Before starting on my path of self-improvement, I had been doing only the minimum I needed to do to provide for my kids, pay the bills, and pass the day—*that* was a rut. Now, getting up in the morning and looking forward to my daily routine—exercising with a friend, writing motivational material, corresponding with those on the path of self-improvement, sharing comments about weight loss on a live chat, reading at night—keeps me enthusiastic. On any given day you will find me doing most or all of these actions, and there is still plenty of variety in my day. Different exercises and topics keep things interesting and in an exciting "zone" rather than a rut. A solid routine comes from knowing where you're going. So define your goals, plan your actions, and develop your daily habits for success.

6. BUILD FAITH AND CONFIDENCE—
ONE ACTION AT A TIME

When I hear someone tell me about the obstacles she faces and her feelings of being overwhelmed, I tell her not to focus on swallowing the elephant whole (an apt metaphor, huh?). The solution is to take one bite at a time when trying to eat the whole elephant. To succeed in any weight-loss effort or at any goal, if you can just decide to take one action that would move you closer to where you want to go, you're on your way. Don't try to take a big leap, because the pain will be great if you fall. You can almost guarantee yourself success when you move ahead one stable and strong step at a time. Taking one action, like substituting fruit for junk food or unhealthy snacks, and doing it for a week at a time, can and should boost your confidence and faith in yourself. Do it for a day and feel good; do it for a week and feel great. Imagine what just one short year will bring.

7. BE RICH WITH KNOWLEDGE, HAPPINESS, AND SPIRIT

Never once in my years of being 130 pounds overweight did I realize that the greatest thing about life *is* life. I didn't know the blessing of having the opportunity to enjoy so many different things. Knowing this has allowed me to find happiness within. I always thought happiness would come only when the scale dictated that it was time. Don't let any amount of weight keep you from being happy. There are plenty of reasons to be happy, and setting out to get healthy and fit will just be icing on the cake (as long as it's not icing *from* the cake).

By finding riches in the knowledge that you have (to be and achieve whatever you want), in the happiness that exists within you (that keeps you positive and healthy), and in your spirit (that will keep you forever strong), you will never again doubt that each day, good or bad, *is* a success, because you were given the chance to *experience* life. Don't let anyone take away your riches, but be sure to use your riches to help others.

8. NEVER FORGET WHERE YOU CAME FROM

Remembering the days when you desired health, you wanted to be fit, your every intention was to start on a diet tomorrow, only to become more frustrated, will help you avoid going backward. I don't often think about or dwell on the pain and misery I felt during that period of my life, but I will never forget. When I find myself wanting a piece of cake or reaching for a cheese appetizer, I often remember a time when reaching for food was all I did, and nine out of ten times I now opt for the sorbet or the veggie platter. If you have started, if you are making consistent progress toward living more healthfully each day, be happy that you are not back at "square one," even if you've just started. Live one day at a time, and, as you begin to take control of your life, don't forget the painful days you are leaving behind. Those will make the happy days you are creating now and in the future that much better!

PART VI

When One Door Closes . . .

You've read about how my life took an unexpected turn. It suddenly became clear to me that I was going to be on my own and therefore needed to get healthy and strong so that I could care for my two children, and my own needs. My marriage needed to end, which was certainly sad; I don't think anyone is really happy when something doesn't work out as it was intended. I allowed that door in my life to close, and I began to look for something new to learn, a way to grow from the experience. I didn't like what and who I had become, not because I was overweight, but because I had let myself become a person with no joy or passion. I did not realize the depth of my unhappiness at the time, but I can clearly see it in hindsight. I took awhile just to get myself and my thoughts together. I went from being extremely depressed to being angry. After a while, this anger allowed me to harness the energy to get moving toward something better. I looked within for strength, and each day I made small steps in the direction I wanted to head.

We all have situations that arise in our lives that upset us, but if you allow anger to remain, it eats you up inside and can cause health problems. As anger faded, I became sad. I was tired of people feeling sorry for me, and, more important, I was sick of feeling sorry for myself. Self-pity is not a healthy emotion; it is a shallow attempt to garner attention for yourself, and it does no one any good, least of all the person feeling it. So don't wallow in self-pity for long. The longer you do, the harder it is to stop.

Eventually I began to rise above the anger and sadness into more constructive and healthy emotions. I am glad I did. Like my dad told me, "It was time to get my house in order." He didn't mean the unfinished construction mess-of-a-house that the kids and I were living in, he meant me—spiritually, emotionally, and, of great concern to him, physically.

I made the decision to change. Because *you* decide you are not going to allow life to get any worse, it then has to get better. I believe that any situation presents two choices: Improve the situation or allow it to worsen. I chose to improve. That was it, the end of the downward spiral. I looked back and knew that I had used many years of life doing things that I couldn't be proud of—and realizing that helped motivate me upward.

I realized that if I didn't change, the misery would only get worse. Realize, as I did, that *you* are far more important than the food you eat. If you understand that now, if you admit the pain that a few, or hundreds, of pounds are causing you, you will be able to get started. In other words, *don't waste any more time of your life!* Time is running out, so make every day count.

Once I decided it was time to treat my body like a temple, like my best friend, by feeding it wonderful, healthy food and caring for it in the best manner possible, I was on my way. The first move I made was to completely swear off my enemy or "vice": ice cream. To this day I won't eat it, and it isn't difficult anymore, but it wasn't easy at first. I did crave ice cream, but I convinced myself that it was to blame for my unhappiness. I made myself come to hate it rather than keeping on hating myself for eating it. I do not feel deprived. I realize that giving in to an unhealthy life deprives me of optimal health. This attitude put my mind back in control. Food stopped being my life. We have to eat to live, not live to eat.

In the past I would start thinking about lunch at ten o'clock: where I would go, what I would order. It's no wonder I couldn't lose weight. Food filled my every thought—well, not every thought: Going on a diet and losing weight was also heavily on my mind.

Looking back, I can see now why I always believed I was dieting and eating healthfully: because I put so much thought and effort into it. If desire or obsession meant anything, I would have been thin long before. Once I quit dwelling on what I would eat, life got a lot easier. I started bringing enough food for the week to the office on Monday and put it in the fridge. At 11:30 A.M. each day, I'd go to the kitchen in my office and make my veggie sandwich and eat—a simple process that didn't require a great deal of thought. The guys at work nicknamed my lunch staple (veggie sandwich) the "stinky sandwich" because, when heated in the microwave, the broccoli and Swiss cheese smelled strong. Smelly, maybe, but it sure tasted great—and it still does! My veggie sandwich is a standard lunch for me, one I eat at least once a week. A surprising result of this one change was that all of the time that I used to spend thinking of food was now freed up, allowing me to spend more time performing my job. My productivity went up by 30 percent *and* I was losing weight.

Another thing I did might be fun for you, too. I recruited others in my office who were interested in healthy eating and formed a healthy-lunch club. Each day one person was responsible for bringing enough lunch to feed themselves as well as the others in the group. It was a lot of fun, and it enabled me to try new recipes and get to know my co-workers better.

Dinner was easy because that wasn't the time of day when I was the hungriest. Worn out after a long day and rushing home to cook for everyone else, I didn't have the appetite I did at other times throughout the day. Usually I'd have a serving of the vegetables and fruit I had prepared for my kids, adding brown rice or pasta. Once or twice a week I splurged on a fresh-veggie pizza (most large supermarkets have one they make fresh daily) with little or no cheese. Later in the evening, if munchies became a problem I would eat, but what I chose to eat was different from what I had chosen in the past. Gone were the gallons of ice cream. Now if I had to eat at night I would reach for bran cereal, fruit, or veggies.

A great food item I recently discovered and I would highly recommend is Gardenburger veggie patties. If you are like me and love the whole hamburger "experience," these are for you. They are meatless patties, low in fat, all natural, and they have a bunch of great flavors—my favorites are the Savory Mushroom and the Veggie Medley. (You should be able to find them in the frozen-food section of most grocery stores.)

On the weekends, something I loved to do was to make a tray of grapes, light crackers, and some good low-fat pâté and leave it around to nibble, like at a cocktail party. I even put my sparkling water in a crystal wineglass. Just because I was alone didn't mean I couldn't live in style. Setting a luxurious mood made me feel that I was treating myself to the best in life, for me and for my body. I would place fresh flowers on the table, use pretty dishes, play some classical music while we dined. Doing so made each time the kids and I were together memorable, and it lessened the feeling that someone or something was missing. Making meals an experience, not just shoveling down food, will raise your appreciation for treating yourself well. The atmosphere should be more the focus and more enjoyable than the food.

Do what I did while losing my weight and still do each day now: Prepare an evening meal for the entire family. Start with a salad with leafy greens, great vegetables, a low-calorie dressing, perhaps a slice of multigrain bakery bread, and a large glass of iced tea or water. While giving thanks, let everyone take turns saying what they are thankful for about their day. Listen to what made everyone's day special or, if you are alone, reflect on what gifts you had that day, and those to look forward to. Focus on spending "quality time" with your loved ones. It is a great time for really finding out what goes on in your kids' lives. Move on to the next course—lean meat, steamed vegetables, a small potato perhaps.

After dinner, enjoy fresh seasonal fruit, and *occasionally* have a treat, maybe angel food cake or pumpkin pie (although I usually recommend that if you eat any treats, you do so in the middle of the day so you have the rest of the day to burn off the "extra fuel"). Healthy menus like these are great not only for you, but for your family, too. I love it when women tell me they can't make a "healthy" meal because they "have to cook for their whole family, not just themselves." I used to make the same comment before I had my awakening.

Stop and think about that comment: Are you the *only* one who deserves to eat healthfully? Are your children or your spouse any less deserving of healthy bodies and a longer life? Just think, everyone will benefit from your healthy lifestyle and the new you. Plus, you'll instill healthy eating habits in your children that will carry them through life. Will they complain and fight you initially when you introduce grilled chicken instead of nuggets fried in lard? Of course! But they also fight about bedtime, toothbrushing, and getting shots. You wouldn't back down from your insistence on these vital points, would you? After a few weeks of meals together it will be much more about being together as a family than about the food you are eating. Meals will be so "Norman Rockwell" you won't believe it.

Simple eating habits made it easy for me to take my mind off eating and focus on other things. This caused me to reflect on other areas of my life that needed attention. So many areas of my life suffered from my being overweight, either directly or indirectly; I knew that I needed to change many things. So first it was a matter of simplifying my eating habits because I needed time and energy to pull other areas of my life together. Only later did I realize that this was the same thinking that allowed me to enjoy my life: For the first time in years, I was focusing on life rather than pleasing myself with food.

When some people hear my weight-loss story they say, "Sure, you lost the weight because of the divorce," forgetting the fact that I lost a great deal of weight prior to separating. No, the Julia I was then would have eaten her way out of a funk. I took what was, to say the least, an emotionally very low point in my life and chose to better myself. It was a compilation of many things that gave me the motivation to change, but the decision and commitment were the keys to getting on the road that would forever change my life. I created a better life for my children and for myself.

I know people who, after an extramarital affair was disclosed, have let the misfortune in their lives consume them. They allow their feelings of devastation to cloud over their lives and often funnel their energies into nonproductive channels. I didn't fall apart, but instead took charge of my life. I had spent years allowing the negative in my life to rule my actions, making me a very negative person. When I truly believed it couldn't get any worse, I knew I needed to change.

We all need something to jump-start our engines, but we have to supply our own fuel. You can be your own energy. There is no better feeling on earth than to face those who have hurt you, hold your head up high, and say, "Look at me now. I'm a survivor. I'm strong and I love me!" It may be hard to imagine feeling that way, but you will. You'll become a larger *being* than you ever were when you were fat.

I share with you the intimate and sad details in my life to show you a light, a ray of hope. No matter what you are dealing with, you can see that change is at hand. You are in control and you can come out on top—accept nothing less than that from yourself. Losing weight is a by-product of self-improvement. Self-Improvement through Self-Motivation will certainly make your waistline thinner, but it will not stop there—it truly will improve every aspect of your life!

Weight loss through my basic principles is a synergistic process. The better you look, the better you feel. The more you consume healthy foods, the better your body will feel and look. This reinforces your positive attitude. People will begin to notice that something is different about you. I started to feel great, and soon craved only (or at least mostly) healthy foods. My body's response became the best motivation I could have asked for. I added a little exercise to get those endorphins flowing, and soon there was no stopping me.

Before long, none of my old clothes fit. Unfortunately, a new wardrobe costs money, so I borrowed a sewing machine from a friend and ran a big seam up the back of all my clothes as they started to get baggy on me. I realize that it may not be in the best professional taste to have a three-inch seam down the back of your dress, but it will make you so proud of yourself and your weight loss. I wore those seams like medals. I showed everyone and proudly told them, "Look—I had to take this in three inches!" Keep going until you reach your goal. Make some new clothes your reward for each new goal reached.

Thrift shops are another good alternative. You can purchase inexpensive skirts, blouses, slacks, and sweaters that can be donated back when you're ready to buy clothes in your "ideal" size. Once you get going on the changes I've suggested, the pounds will melt off so quickly that by this season next year you will need a new wardrobe. I went from a size twenty-two to a size eight to ten, and sometimes a six. You may not be able to imagine it today, but I promise you, if you eat healthy foods prepared in a healthy way, avoid sweets, drink water, and get exercise, you will improve your body and your life.

Change is never easy, but it is possible, and it's much easier if you stick to the basic principles given here. You have to want it. And you have to want to avoid the negative aspect of refusing to change. Something needs to get you going from behind, and something needs to pull you forward: the carrot-and-stick theory.

Each day make the decision to live a healthy life and commit yourself to achieving it. Make it your goal, make it your dream. A wise man once told me, "Make no small dreams, for there is no magic in them." You need to see that living a full, healthy, and complete life does have a certain amount of magic about it! Look at children. Everything they do is fun, so full of life, so in awe of it, so full of magic. Just because we are older doesn't mean we can't live our lives with those same elements of magic and awe. Magic is so positive, so energizing. Life is an adventure and is meant to be lived that way. What a boring existence to have your days revolve around what food to eat and what is on television. Soon a magical life will become second nature, ingrained in your thoughts. Remind yourself daily that achieving your goal will feel a lot better (for a lot longer) than the unhealthy food will taste. Going to the park with your kids or hiking will provide you with memories that will last a lot longer than what happened on your favorite show. Make yourself believe that you are special, much more than a body with too much food in it.

Here are a few of my daily guidelines that have helped me to stay on the path of Self-Improvement through Self-Motivation:

- **Stay off the scale.** The primary role of exercise is to burn calories but, at the same time, you are reshaping your body with muscle tissue that weighs more than fat tissue. Use your measurements, the way your clothes fit (even a body-fat analysis) as ways to evaluate your progress as well as your maintenance. Remember, you're not on a diet and the scale is only one measure of your success. It matters much more to me how I look than what I weigh.

- **Exercise your cardiovascular system.** Three to five days each week for twenty to sixty minutes using activities like walking, biking, stair climbing, cross-country skiing, swimming, or circuit training with weights is a good beginning goal. To increase fat loss, build up to sixty minutes a day at a moderate pace. The "talk test" is a good indicator of intensity. It requires that you work out at a level that still allows you to talk or carry on a conversation comfortably during your activity. If you can't talk, you're not working out effectively.

- **Include strength training two or three days a week in your exercise routine to shape muscles and build lean body mass.** Increasing muscle tissue raises your metabolism, making it easier to maintain your new weight. The craze in weight loss these days is building muscle mass—the more you have, the better your body burns calories! Anaerobic exercise (strength training with weights) burns 500 percent more calories than aerobic exercise. Do it now!

- **Use it or lose it.** Muscle tissue does not turn to fat once you stop training, but your body needs to be active. (I don't know why or when you will "stop" training—you don't want to gain the fat back, do you?) The body requires maintenance, just like your car. The big difference, of course, is that you can abuse your car and trade it in for a new one.

- **Establish a workout schedule and stick to it, making it a habit.** Find the time of day that best fits your schedule. If there is no time available in your schedule, you need to rearrange your priorities. Exercise is an essential component of your new habits and lifestyle. Scheduling workout times on your calendar can help you to squeeze exercise into your busy day. You can seek the help of a personal trainer just to establish a routine and a commitment to stick with it.

- **Set a long-term, six-month goal for yourself.** Then break that down into short-term, weekly goals. For example, a long-term goal could be dropping two jeans sizes. Your short-term goal may be to walk (or use the treadmill) three miles by the second week (not stopping until you reach that point), and cross-training with weights three days a week. By the way, if you are exercising at home and walking, use your car to measure the distance in order for you to get the correct mileage (be sure it's a round trip!).

- **Set realistic goals.** A trainer can help establish a healthy weight for you based upon your height, frame size, age, and body composition. With most everything, you can set your own goals and reach them if you put your mind to it. But as for the body, weight loss at an accelerated pace is *not* healthy, and it could be dangerous. Your body will be good to you if you are good to it. Fill out your goal sheet and stick to it.

- **Reward yourself for small accomplishments along the way.** Remember, I used the manicure, massage, and many other services available at the salon and spa in my town. The many fabulous services at a spa and salon are a great way of rewarding yourself for reaching goals.

- **Have fun with your exercise.** This is not a prison sentence! Realistically, you need to include exercise in your lifestyle forever, so have some fun with it. Try new activities, take a class, listen to fun music, share your time with a buddy, or, as I did, see how much you can make your trainer laugh during the workout to keep her or him entertained and losing count of your sit-ups.

- **Live a healthy lifestyle.** Managing your weight is best accomplished through changes in lifestyle, habits, and attitude—the foundation of getting on the road to health. The foundation of your new lifestyle involves things that are fun, alive, energetic, and inspiring. You will throw out some of the old habits and replace them with things you may never have considered. This can be a bit overwhelming at times, so it helps to surround yourself with a network of people who can support you, coach you, and motivate you to be your best. Most important, these people should be positive, focused, and getting the most out of life, which you want to do, too.

Discipline yourself by following these guidelines and you will excel!

PART VII

Eating Plans

One-Week Menu Plan

DAY 1

Breakfast:
1 Easy Egg Omelette (page 189)
1 cup yogurt, low-fat, any flavor
1 serving fruit
1 cup skim milk

Lunch:
Veggie Sandwich (page 207)
1 cup mini carrots, raw
1 cup red grapes

Snack:
Bagel, 2 tbsp. peanut butter

Dinner:
Grilled Tuna (page 256)
Herb-Grilled Vegetables (page 228)
1 cup cooked brown rice
1 serving fruit

DAY 2

Breakfast:
Whole-Wheat Pancakes (pages 194-195), 2 tbsp. light syrup
2 servings fruit
1 cup skim milk

Lunch:

Gardenburger Fire-Roasted Focaccia (pages 220–221)

1 rice cake

1 serving fruit

Snack:

3 cups light microwave popcorn

Dinner:

Beef Tenderloin Delight (page 236)

Stuffed Mushrooms (pages 215–216)

2 cups mixed-greens salad, 2 tbsp. dressing

DAY 3

Breakfast:

Banana Milk Smoothie (pages 186-187)

Whole-wheat bagel, 2 tbsp. peanut butter

Lunch:

Vegetable Pizza (page 206)

1 serving fruit

Snack:

1 Healthy Choice fat-free granola bar

1 cup skim milk

Dinner:

Shrimp Kabobs (page 248)

Marinated Vegetables (pages 219–220)

2 cups mixed-greens salad

DAY 4

Breakfast:

Breakfast Sandwich (page 194)

1 serving fruit

Lunch:

Grilled Chicken Caesar Salad (page 196)

4 crackers or baked wontons sprinkled with Parmesan

1 serving fruit

Snack:

Bunch of red grapes, small wedge of Cheddar cheese, 2 crackers

Dinner:

Broccoli Chicken (page 247)

Creamy Cucumbers (page 219)

⅓ cup Chinese noodles

1 serving fruit

DAY 5

Breakfast:

Vegetable Omelette (page 191)

English muffin, 1 tsp. honey

2 servings fruit

Lunch:

Nutty Spinach Salad (page 197)

1 small roll

1 serving fruit

Snack:

Carrots, celery, and cauliflower cuts—unlimited

Dinner:

Italian Zucchini Bowls (page 226)

2 cups romaine lettuce, 1 tbsp. Parmesan cheese, sliced red onions, artichoke hearts, diced roasted red pepper, and light Italian dressing

Summer Risotto (pages 257–258)

DAY 6

Breakfast:
Oatmeal and Fruit (page 192)

Lunch:
Easy Tuna Salad (page 212)
2 hard-boiled eggs, whites only
1 whole-wheat pita
1 serving fruit

Snack:
3 cups light microwave popcorn

Dinner:
Swordfish Steak (pages 253–254)
Glazed Carrots (page 222)
2 cups salad

DAY 7

Breakfast:
Egg Burrito (page 193)
2 servings fruit

Lunch:
Rice with Herbs (pages 213–214)
Carrots
1 serving fruit

Snack:
5 graham crackers
1 cup skim milk

Dinner:
Chicken Breasts with Pesto (page 241)
Parmesan Veggies (page 220)
2 cups salad, mixed veggies
Angel Food Cake (page 266)

Recipes

Many of my recipes are for one serving unless otherwise noted. The breakfast and lunch recipes are individual servings, and the dinners are for a family. I cook for my family and developed these for the whole family; my children and husband all eat and like these healthy recipes.

If you are cooking for many, you can adjust the recipe to accommodate more, or make a bigger batch and freeze some for another time if you are cooking for only one and want to save time. I do not focus on the calorie count, numbers of grams of fat, or nutritional value of my recipes. That would not be in keeping with my belief that food is fuel and therefore not to be obsessed about. These recipes were and still are staples of my daily food intake. They helped me to lose 130 pounds and to keep it off for many years. These are healthy, hearty, and tasty foods. As with any "diet," please be sure to check with your health-care provider and make sure he or she gives the green light for you to switch to these and other healthy foods. I am sure you will love my recipes, but they need not be all that you ever eat again. Let common sense and good health be your guides.

MORNING EYE-OPENERS

The following are a few healthy drinks I like to use in the morning. There are many, many variations on these types of drinks. There are a couple of things I like to use consistently when making a morning drink. One is whey protein, one of the best sources of protein. The second is wheat germ, which is an excellent source of fiber. You will also see that bananas are a recurring ingredient; they are high in potassium and have many great health benefits. You can use many different fruit combinations and variations that suit your taste. By keeping to low-fat yogurt, non-fat milk, and banana as a base, you can avoid that strong acidic taste. This keeps the drink from being too hard on your stomach if you have a sensitive digestive system. Also, you can add any of your favorite extracts to the smoothies—almond, vanilla, and the like. For those of you who like to have coffee in the morning, you can put a small amount of cold coffee in the smoothie. (A *small* amount of caffeine can help burn calories.) The smoothies are all single-serving recipes.

Fruit Smoothie

1 cup vanilla low-fat yogurt
½ cup each skim milk and orange juice
⅓ cup each sliced frozen peaches, blueberries, strawberries
¼ cup ice
1 or 2 scoops protein powder (optional)

Put all ingredients in blender and chop until ice is crushed thoroughly. With a scoop or two of protein powder, this smoothie makes a great morning meal. The kids even love it. If you're going to exercise, this will help fuel your body to get the fat burning, as will any of these smoothies.

Serves one.

Banana Milk Smoothie

1 banana
1 cup skim milk

½ cup ice
½ tsp. vanilla extract
1 scoop protein powder (optional)

Put everything in the blender and set on Crush for approximately 30 seconds until the contents become a thick liquid. Add more milk to thin if too thick. Of course a scoop of protein powder can be added for a source of protein.

Serves one.

MULTI-FRUIT SMOOTHIE

1 banana
1 kiwi
1 lime
1 cup skim milk
½ 6-oz. can frozen orange-juice concentrate
½ cup ice
1 tbsp. honey
1 packet Revival soy vanilla protein power

Combine all ingredients in a blender and set on Crush for approximately 30 seconds until the mixture becomes a thick liquid. Add milk as necessary to thin.

Serves one.

BREAKFAST SMOOTHIE

½ cup skim milk
¼ cup vanilla non-fat yogurt
¼ cup ice
1 or 2 egg whites
½ tsp. vanilla extract

Combine all ingredients in a blender and blend until mixture is smooth.

Serves one.

Banana and Yogurt Smoothie

1 cup plain non-fat yogurt
½ cup orange juice
½ cup favorite fruit
1 banana
¼ cup ice
1 tbsp. wheat germ

Put ingredients in a blender and blend until mixture is smooth.

Serves one.

Tropical Smoothie

1½ cups non-fat milk
1 cup mango or papaya sorbet
1 or 2 bananas
¼ cup pineapple and/or kiwi
¼ cup ice
2 tbsp. whey protein

Put ingredients in a blender and blend until mixture is smooth.

Serves one.

TROPICAL SHAKE

1½ cups vanilla low-fat yogurt
1 cup sliced frozen peaches
¾ cup non-fat milk
⅓ cup ice
¼ cup strawberries or blueberries
¼ cup frozen orange-juice concentrate
1 tbsp. wheat germ
1 tsp. almond extract

Combine all ingredients in a blender and crush until smooth.

Serves one.

QUICK BREAKFAST

Shredded Wheat cereal with non-fat milk
1 banana
1 8-oz. cup hot tea

Serves one.

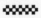

EASY EGG OMELETTE

3 cherry tomatoes, chopped
2 or 3 egg whites
Water

Put cherry tomatoes in a skillet on medium heat. Beat egg whites and add to the skillet. Put a small amount (1 teaspoon) of water in the skillet and cover. This will, in effect, steam the eggs. Remove when the texture is lightly hardened. Serve with fruit and a cup of tea or non-fat milk.

Serves one.

CREAM OF WHEAT

¾ cup water
¾ cup non-fat milk
Salt
⅓ cup Cream of Wheat
1 tbsp. wheat germ
2 tbsp. honey
¼ tsp. ground nutmeg

In a medium saucepan, put water, milk, and salt on medium high, then stir in Cream of Wheat and bring to a boil, stirring occasionally and more frequently as mixture begins to boil. When the desired thickness is attained, take pan off the heat, stir in wheat germ, and let stand. When still warm, put into a serving bowl and add honey and nutmeg. This is a good healthy way to start the day.

Serves one.

OAT MUFFINS

2 cups Quaker Oat Bran hot cereal, uncooked
⅓ cup plus 1 tbsp. brown sugar
¼ cup whole-wheat flour
2 tsp. baking powder
¼ tsp. salt
¼ tsp. nutmeg
2 egg whites, beaten
1 cup non-fat milk
3 tbsp. light vegetable oil
1 tsp. vanilla extract
¼ cup Quaker Oats

Preheat oven to 400°. Line muffin tins with paper baking cups. Combine oat bran cereal, ⅓ cup brown sugar, flour, baking powder, salt, and nutmeg. In a separate bowl combine egg whites, milk, oil, and vanilla and mix. Add to first bowl and mix well. Fill baking cups almost full. Put oats and 1 tablespoon brown sugar in a small bowl and mix. Spread over almost-full cups. Bake for 20 minutes. Serve with fruit.

One muffin per serving. Makes twelve.

Vegetable Omelette

3 egg whites, beaten
2 small mushrooms
1 cherry tomato, chopped
1 tbsp. chopped yellow onion
Dash freshly ground black pepper
Sprinkle of low-fat cheese

Combine all ingredients, except cheese, in a skillet over medium heat. Sprinkle on a small amount of your choice of low-fat cheese. Serve with one slice of whole-wheat toast and a ten-ounce glass of non-fat milk. This is a classic omelette that is great any morning.

Serves one.

Multi-Vegetable Omelette

4 egg whites
¼ cup chopped vegetables (zucchini, mushroom, green onion, green pepper, cherry tomato)
1 tsp. olive oil
¼ tsp. (fresh or dried) basil
Dash salt and freshly ground black pepper

Beat egg whites in a small bowl. Add chopped vegetables to a skillet that has been coated with oil on medium heat. After 1 or 2 minutes, add egg whites, along with basil and salt and pepper and cover, cooking slowly. Fold omelette in half when almost completely cooked. Serve when center is no longer runny. Serve with a slice of whole-wheat toast and a glass of non-fat milk or warm tea.

Serves one.

Eggs on the Go

2 hard-boiled eggs, leave out 1 yolk
Fruit plate w/cantaloupe and honeydew
1 slice whole-wheat toast
1 glass non-fat milk or tea

Hard-boiled eggs are quick and easy if you're on the go. Taking out one or both yolks keeps the fat content low. Make a dozen hard-boiled eggs and keep them available for breakfast or a quick snack in the afternoon.

Serves one.

Oatmeal and Fruit

Oatmeal
Water
1 tsp. almond or vanilla extract
Cinnamon (optional)

Cook one serving of oatmeal in water, following directions on package. (Avoid using the pre-measured individual packages; they are high in sugar.) Add almond or vanilla extract for flavor, or sprinkle with cinnamon instead. Serve with fresh fruit on the side—bananas, grapefruit, or an apple—and with a cup of coffee or tea.

Serves one.

ASPARAGUS-MUSHROOM OMELETTE

2 large egg whites
½ tsp. minced chives
1 tsp. water
Dash salt and freshly ground black pepper
1 tsp. unsalted butter
1 tbsp. chopped asparagus
3 large mushroom caps, chopped
2 slices tomato, chopped
1 tbsp. minced parsley

Whisk together egg whites, chives, water, and salt and pepper in a medium-size bowl. Melt butter in medium skillet over medium-high heat. Add asparagus and mushrooms, cooking and stirring for a minute. Turn heat down to medium low, add egg mixture, and cover, cooking slowly. Check after a minute, and fold omelette over. Remove when no longer runny. Top with tomato and sprinkle with parsley.

Serves one.

EGG BURRITO

3 egg whites, beaten
1 tsp. water
½ oz. low-fat Cheddar (or other) cheese
1 fat-free wheat tortilla
½ oz. salsa

Place egg whites in a skillet over medium heat. Add water and cover for 3 minutes. This will steam the eggs. Add eggs and cheese to the tortilla, along with salsa, and roll it up. Serve with a fruit bowl and a glass of non-fat milk.

Serves one.

BREAKFAST SANDWICH

3 egg whites
2 slices whole-wheat bread, toasted
1 tbsp. low-fat cream cheese
1 tsp. apricot fruit spread
1 slice low-fat, low-salt ham
1 large lettuce leaf

Beat egg whites. Cook in a nonstick skillet. On one toasted slice of bread, spread cream cheese. On other slice, spread fruit spread. Add egg whites, slice of ham, and lettuce to make a sandwich. Serve with a glass of non-fat milk or a cup of tea.

Serves one.

OPEN-FACED BAGEL SANDWICH

1 whole-wheat or nine-grain bagel
Fat-free (or low-fat) cream cheese
2 slices red onion
2 slices smoked fish (salmon is my favorite)
2 slices tomato
1 tsp. capers

Lightly toast the bagel. Spread a small amount of cream cheese on each bagel half. Put an onion slice, then a fish slice, then a tomato slice on each half. Sprinkle with capers. This is a great meal that will satisfy any appetite. Serve with a glass of non-fat milk or a cup of tea.

Serves one.

WHOLE-WHEAT PANCAKES

1 cup buttermilk
1 egg

4 tsp. vegetable oil
1 tbsp. firmly packed brown sugar
1 cup whole-wheat flour
1 cup rolled oats
1 tsp. double-acting baking powder
½ tsp. baking soda
½ tsp. salt

In a medium mixing bowl combine buttermilk, egg, oil, and sugar, and beat until thoroughly mixed. Add remaining ingredients, stirring until smooth. Pour small portions into a hot non-stick skillet. Cook on each side until brown.

I put this recipe here because it was given to me a couple of years ago by a relative and it is great. If you are crunched for time, the easy way to make whole-wheat pancakes is to buy whole-wheat pancake mix (non-fat if possible), and prepare with water. Serve with fruit.

Two pancakes per serving. Makes six.

LUNCH LIGHTS

Lunch is a time to eat something that keeps your energy and blood-sugar levels from dropping too much, but you don't want to make it a meal that will weigh you down. Too many times I find that people are eating a big lunch that makes them tired and groggy in the afternoon. Productivity in the workplace actually slows down because of the meals that are eaten at the noon hour. If you want to keep your energy levels high and your metabolism operating efficiently, eat smart. The meals I have outlined here are just that—smart, healthy, light meals. Remember to keep things simple. During my 130-pound weight loss, and still today, I keep all my meals simple. Let your meals be just an action you take to provide your body with nutrition, not an event of pleasure that could cause you pain later. Eat to live, don't live to eat. This is simply the fuel for your body that lets you live an active life.

Note: Many of the salads are great for dinner, too.

GRILLED CHICKEN CAESAR SALAD

1 cup romaine or any dark, leafy lettuce
1 tbsp. light Caesar dressing (low-fat preferable)
4 or 5 cherry tomatoes, sliced
1 slice red onion, chopped
1 hard-boiled egg (white only), chopped
1 grilled skinless, boneless chicken breast
Dash crushed red pepper
1 tbsp. lemon juice

Tear lettuce into pieces in a large bowl. Add dressing, tomatoes, onion, and egg and toss. Add chicken. Add crushed red pepper to taste, and squeeze lemon juice over salad. This is great with a glass of iced tea.

Serves one.

SPINACH AND PINE NUT SALAD

2 tsp. olive oil
2 tsp. pine nuts
2 tsp. raisins
¼ clove garlic, chopped
2 cups trimmed fresh spinach
Salt and freshly ground black pepper to taste

In a small skillet, heat 1 teaspoon oil on medium heat, then add 1 teaspoon nuts and 1 teaspoon raisins, cooking until golden brown. Remove and set aside. Add 1 teaspoon oil and the garlic with half of the spinach to the same pan, sprinkling salt and pepper modestly. Cook until spinach wilts, about 1 to 2 minutes. Put in a bowl. Add remaining spinach to pan and sprinkle with salt and pepper, heating as before. Take out and combine all mixtures in the bowl, and add remaining nuts and raisins. Toss. This can be prepared ahead of time and taken to work for lunch.

Serves one.

Nutty Spinach Salad

½ cup walnuts
4 tbsp. blue cheese
1 tbsp. honey
1 16-oz. bag fresh spinach
4 chicken breasts, broiled and cut up
½ cup chopped mushrooms
½ red onion, sliced
Dash freshly ground black pepper
Spinach salad dressing (low-fat)

Place walnuts on a piece of foil and sprinkle with blue cheese, drizzle with honey, and broil lightly for 2 or 3 minutes. Place washed spinach in a bowl and add chicken, mushrooms, onion, and pepper and toss. Add walnut mix and a few tablespoons of dressing. (I like T. Marzetti's spinach dressing, which is fattening, so use sparingly.) Toss and serve.

Serves four.

Fruit Salad with Almonds

1 cup romaine lettuce
1 cup fresh spinach
¼ cup halved grapes
¼ cup mandarin oranges
2 tbsp. salad oil
1 tbsp. wine vinegar
¼ clove garlic, minced
1 tbsp. brown sugar
1 tsp. minced chives
1 tsp. curry powder
Dash soy sauce
¼ cup almonds
¼ avocado, sliced

Tear lettuce and spinach and combine with grapes and oranges. Combine oil, vinegar, garlic, brown sugar, chives, curry powder, and soy sauce in a small bowl and stir vigorously. Pour this dressing over the greens and toss. Almonds should be broiled in the oven for 1 to 3 minutes to toast. Add almonds and avocado.

Serves two.

Papaya Salad

1 small peeled orange, cut into bite-size pieces
1 ripe papaya, cut into bite-size pieces
½ grapefruit, cut into bite-size pieces
2 or 3 thin slices red onion
2 thin slices red and yellow pepper, quartered

Combine all ingredients in a bowl. Prepare the following dressing:

1 tsp. lime juice
1 tsp. olive oil
¼ tsp. Dijon-style mustard

Combine in a small bowl and mix thoroughly. Add to salad and toss. This is great to prepare in the morning to take to work. Put the dressing in a separate container until ready to serve. Great with a glass of iced tea.

Serves one.

GARDEN VINAIGRETTE SALAD

1 grilled skinless, boneless chicken breast, cut up
1 cup romaine or other dark lettuce
¼ cup cauliflower, broken into small pieces
¼ cup sliced zucchini
4 cherry tomatoes, each cut in half
2 tbsp. chopped yellow onion
1 tbsp. vinaigrette dressing (low- or non-fat)

Grill or broil the chicken the night before, and then you can have it ready for tomorrow's lunch. Put all the ingredients in a bowl and toss. Have a slice of whole-wheat bread with your salad, and a tall glass of water or iced tea.

Serves one.

ARTICHOKE AND CHICKEN SALAD

1 grilled skinless, boneless chicken breast, cut up
2 cups romaine or any dark lettuce
¼ cup artichoke hearts, drained and cut
2 tbsp. chopped fresh cilantro
2 tbsp. cider vinegar
1 tbsp. olive oil
½ tsp. dried basil
½ tsp. sugar

If you plan on having this for lunch, preparing the chicken the night before is easier. Or you may want to prepare a couple of chicken breasts for use in the next couple of lunches. Put all the ingredients in a bowl and toss. If you're taking this to work, leave out the oil, vinegar, and artichoke hearts until ready to serve. You can combine these in a separate container until ready to serve.

Serves one.

Light Pasta Salad

4 oz. whole-wheat pasta
6 sun-dried tomatoes, chopped (use dry)
1 tsp. balsamic vinegar
1 tsp. olive oil
1 tsp. minced garlic
1 tsp. freshly ground black pepper
¼ cup chopped scallions
2 tbsp. chopped zucchini
Dash dried basil
Dash grated Parmesan cheese

Cook pasta according to directions. Drain two-thirds of the water and, with pasta still in water, put in sun-dried tomatoes and let soak for 2 minutes. Pour contents into a colander. In a small bowl combine vinegar, oil, garlic, and pepper, and mix with a fork. In your serving bowl combine pasta and tomatoes with the remaining ingredients, then add oil mixture and toss. You can sprinkle on some Parmesan to taste. This is a great lunch with excellent nutritional value. To take to work, keep the oil mixture separate until ready to serve.

Serves one.

Cilantro Caesar

2 cups romaine or any dark lettuce
4 cherry tomatoes, cut in half
2 fresh scallions, thinly sliced
1 tbsp. minced cilantro
2 tsp. fat-free Caesar dressing
1 tsp. lemon juice
1 tsp. grated Parmesan cheese

Combine all ingredients except lemon juice and Parmesan in a bowl and toss. Then add lemon juice and Parmesan to taste.

Serves one.

Vegetable Salad

1 16-oz. can cut green beans, drained
1 16-oz. can cut wax beans, drained
1 16-oz. can diced carrots, drained
½ cup chopped celery
⅓ cup vinegar
¼ cup sugar
2 tbsp. salad oil
½ tsp. salt
½ tsp. freshly ground black pepper

Combine all vegetables in a bowl. Combine everything else in a small bowl and mix. Pour marinade over vegetables and toss. Cover and let marinate for 2 hours or overnight. Drain off oil and serve. Great for lunch or a light afternoon snack.

Serves about six.

SPINACH SALAD

2 tbsp. chopped yellow onion
1 tbsp. extra-virgin olive oil
1 tsp. catsup
1 tsp. sugar
1 tsp. balsamic vinegar
Dash salt and freshly ground black pepper
Splash Worcestershire sauce
1 slice bacon
2 cups spinach or romaine lettuce
1 4 oz. can water chestnuts, drained and sliced
1 small carrot, thinly sliced
1 hard-boiled egg white

Put onion in blender with oil, catsup, sugar, vinegar, salt and pepper, and splash of Worcestershire. Blend until smooth. Put into a small bowl or cup and chill. Cook bacon slice and remove as much grease as possible with a paper towel. Place spinach or lettuce in a salad bowl, adding water chestnuts, carrot, and crumbled bacon. Add dressing, along with chopped egg white. Toss and serve.

Serves one.

VEGETABLES AND RICE

1 tsp. extra-virgin olive oil
1 carrot, cut into short strips
1 small yellow onion, chopped
½ cup uncooked white or brown rice
1 cup low-salt chicken broth
1 zucchini, cut into long strips
½ cup chopped broccoli
¼ cup frozen green peas
2 tsp. grated Parmesan cheese

Heat oil in a skillet over medium heat. Cook carrot and onion, stirring until slightly crisp. Stir in rice, stirring frequently until rice begins to brown. Pour in half the broth, stirring until liquid is absorbed, and then cook another 15 to 20 minutes after adding the rest of the broth. When rice is tender and creamy, add all other vegetables and stir. Put in a serving dish, sprinkle on Parmesan, and serve.

Serves one.

SALAD WITH ORANGES AND ALMONDS

1 tsp. minced parsley
1 tsp. balsamic vinegar
1 tsp. extra-virgin olive oil
1 tsp. minced garlic
¼ tsp. sugar
¼ tsp. freshly ground black pepper
1 tsp. water
2 scallions, thinly sliced
1 celery stalk, sliced
2 cups romaine lettuce
½ cup mandarin oranges, drained
1 tbsp. toasted chopped almonds

Combine parsley, vinegar, oil, garlic, sugar, pepper, and water in a small bowl and whisk thoroughly. In your serving bowl combine everything else and toss. Add oil mixture and toss again. A great afternoon delight.

Serves one.

MARINATED VEGGIE MIX

1 8-oz. can green beans, drained and cut
1 8-oz. can wax beans, drained and cut

6 cherry tomatoes
2 fresh carrots, thinly sliced
¼ cup chopped celery
2 tbsp. cider vinegar
2 tbsp. sugar
1 tbsp. salad oil
Dash salt and freshly ground black pepper

Combine vegetables in medium bowl. In separate bowl, mix vinegar, sugar, oil, and salt and pepper. Add mixture to vegetables and toss. Chill for at least two hours. Drain marinade into bowl when ready to serve, and use to sprinkle on veggies.

Serves four.

Healthy Turkey Salad

¼ cup vanilla non-fat yogurt
1 tsp. honey
1 tsp. balsamic vinegar
1 cup romaine lettuce
¼ cup cantaloupe, cut into small pieces
¼ cup halved seedless grapes
¼ cup chopped cooked turkey breast
5 pineapple cubes, halved
1 tbsp. minced fresh mint
1 tbsp. minced fresh parsley
1 tsp. pine nuts
1 tsp. raisins

In a small bowl combine yogurt, honey, and vinegar and whisk. In your serving bowl, combine all other ingredients. Then pour honey mixture over salad and toss. Smart and simple.

Serves one.

Potato Salad

1 small potato
¼ cup plain non-fat yogurt
1 tbsp. chopped green onion
1 tbsp. frozen peas, thawed
1 tbsp. chopped green pepper
1 tbsp. chopped red pepper
1 tsp. minced fresh basil
1 tsp. minced fresh parsley
Dash salt and several dashes of freshly ground black pepper

Cook peeled potato in boiling water until tender. Mix all other ingredients in serving bowl. Cube potato and mix into ingredients. Nice as a lunch or served with meat for dinner.

Serves one.

Special Fruit Salad

1 peach, sliced and cut into small pieces
½ tart apple, cored and chopped
½ orange, peeled, sectioned, and cut
½ cup strawberry halves
1 cup plain non-fat yogurt
1 tsp. brown sugar
¼ tsp. ginger

In a bowl toss all fruit. In a separate small bowl, combine yogurt, brown sugar, and ginger and whisk. Add to fruit and toss. A nice light afternoon treat.

Serves one or two.

Vegetable Pizza

1 pizza dough, uncooked
1 tbsp. chopped yellow onion
3 Roma tomatoes, thinly sliced
¼ cup chopped broccoli
¼ cup sliced carrots
¼ cup sliced mushrooms
¼ cup fat-free Italian dressing
¼ cup shredded reduced-fat mozzarella cheese

Bake pizza dough according to directions. After 3 minutes of baking, spread the onion, then the tomatoes, broccoli, carrots, and mushrooms evenly on dough. Pour dressing evenly on top, then sprinkle mozzarella evenly as well. Put back in oven and bake until golden brown. Half of the pie will suffice as a serving. Enjoy a slice!

Serves two.

Shrimp and Vegetables with Rice

1 tbsp. extra-virgin olive oil
¼ cup chopped green onion
¼ cup chopped mushrooms
½ cup medium, uncooked, peeled, deveined shrimp (thawed if
    frozen)
1 tbsp. fat-free Italian dressing
1 cup cooked brown rice

Heat oil in a non-stick skillet, adding onion and mushrooms. Cook at medium heat, then add shrimp. Add dressing and cover and simmer for 10 minutes. Pour shrimp mix over rice, draining excess liquid before doing so. Serve.

Serves one.

TUNA PITA

¼ 6 oz. can tuna, drained and chopped
¼ cup crumbled feta cheese
2 tbsp. thinly sliced celery
¼ cup diced apples
1 tbsp. chopped walnuts
1 tbsp. (fresh or dried) tarragon
Dash salt and freshly ground black pepper
1 pita bread, halved
4 leaves green lettuce

In a medium mixing bowl, combine tuna, feta, celery, apples, nuts, and tarragon and mix well. Stir in salt and pepper. Line a pita pocket with 2 lettuce leaves, fill with half the tuna mixture. Since this makes two servings you can eat one and save the rest for the next day.

Serves two.

VEGGIE SANDWICH

2 slices nine-grain bread
2 slices green pepper
2 slices red pepper
2 slices tomato
1 slice low-fat Lorraine Swiss cheese
1 cup broccoli slaw

Lightly toast the bread, then stack all the remaining ingredients on a plate and microwave on high for about 2 minutes or cook 2 minutes under a broiler. (Use broiler for best results!) Stack on bread. Let cool slightly and serve.

This is one sandwich I made many times during my weight loss, as my former co-workers will attest. It has a distinct aroma, and they always knew when I was making it. It is a great source of nutrition and fiber. For those who don't know, broccoli slaw is a mixture of shredded broccoli, cabbage, and carrots, plain, with no dressing. I use Mann's prepackaged.

Serves one.

Salsa Gardenburger

1 hamburger-style Gardenburger low-fat patty
1 slice low-fat jalapeño jack cheese
1 leaf green lettuce
1 whole-wheat or multi-grain bun
1 tbsp. salsa

Cook patty as indicated on the package. (I microwave mine.) Top with cheese and allow to melt. Place lettuce on bottom bun, top with patty, add salsa, and enjoy.

I forgo the bun, and I like to add a slice of avocado and have black beans on the side.

Serves one.

Spaghetti Squash

1 spaghetti squash, cut lengthwise and seeded
1 thin zucchini, thinly sliced lengthwise
1 sweet red pepper, thinly sliced lengthwise
1 tsp. olive oil
2 cloves garlic, minced
1 cup cherry tomatoes, halved
1 tbsp. white wine vinegar
1 tbsp. minced fresh basil
2 tsp. minced fresh oregano
¼ tsp. freshly ground black pepper
2 tbsp. grated Parmesan cheese

In order to soften squash, microwave in a microwave-safe bowl, one half at a time, on high for 4 minutes. Let stand for 5 minutes. During that time, sauté zucchini and red pepper in oil for 3 minutes in a large non-stick frying pan over medium-high heat. Stir in garlic and cook for 1 minute. Add tomatoes, vinegar, basil, oregano, and pepper; sauté for 2 minutes. Run two forks across squash, "fluffing" the inside of the squash into strands. Add to the frying pan and sauté for 3 minutes. Sprinkle with Parmesan.

Serves four.

CAVATELLI AND PESTO

⅓ cup fresh spinach leaves, packed
1 tbsp. fresh basil
1 tsp. fresh parsley
1 tbsp. grated Parmesan cheese
1 tbsp. non-fat chicken stock
1 tsp. extra-virgin olive oil
1 tsp. chopped garlic
Dash freshly ground black pepper and red-pepper flakes
4 oz. uncooked cavatelli

Thoroughly chop (almost mince) spinach, basil, and parsley. Then add greens to a bowl with Parmesan, stock, oil, garlic, black pepper, and pepper flakes. Mix thoroughly. Cook cavatelli according to directions. Drain and place in a large bowl. Add the pesto mix and toss. A nice afternoon treat with a glass of iced tea.

Serves one.

GAZPACHO SALAD

1 4-serving envelope low-calorie lemon-flavored gelatin
¾ cup boiling water

¾ cup vegetable juice cocktail
2 tbsp. low-calorie Italian dressing
4 tsp. vinegar
½ cup sliced cauliflower flowerets
½ cup chopped, seeded tomato
½ cup chopped celery
¼ cup chopped green pepper

Dissolve gelatin in boiling water. Stir in vegetable juice cocktail, salad dressing, and vinegar. Chill until partially set (the consistency of unbeaten egg whites). Fold in cauliflower, tomato, celery, and green pepper. Turn into a 3-cup mold. Chill several hours or until firm.

Serves four.

SEAFOOD AND VEGGIE QUICHE

4 low-fat prepared biscuits
8 eggs, 7 yolks removed
8 oz. deveined, chopped shrimp
5 oz. low-fat Lorraine Swiss cheese, shredded
2½ cups cauliflower, boiled until partially cooked
1 cup chopped mushrooms
½ cup minced yellow onion
Dash salt and freshly ground black pepper

Coat a pie dish with non-stick (non-fat) spray. Halve the biscuits, and spread 4 halves on the pie dish. Bake in 325° preheated oven for 5 minutes. Let cool. In a bowl, lightly beat eggs and mix with all other ingredients. Put mixture on partially baked biscuits, then put other biscuit halves evenly on top and bake until filling is set, approximately 40 minutes.

Eat a small portion, as the biscuits can be heavy. You can make variations of this recipe by putting different vegetables into the mix.

This dish keeps for reheating later, or freeze the uneaten portion and serve it for dinner on a busy day.

Serves four.

LASAGNA PRIMAVERA

12 oz. uncooked lasagna noodles
1 15-oz. container light ricotta cheese
2 carrots, shredded
1 large onion, chopped
¼ cup chopped mushrooms
¼ cup chopped Roma tomatoes
¼ cup grated Parmesan cheese
3 egg whites
2 cloves garlic, minced
1 tbsp. olive oil
1 tbsp. Italian seasoning

Prepare noodles according to instructions. Combine all other ingredients and mix thoroughly. Lay out one-third of the noodles in an 8-by-10 ovenproof dish. Spread half of mix on noodles. Cover mix with half of remaining noodles. Spread other half of mix on this layer, then cover with remainder of noodles. Bake at 350° for 30 minutes or until golden brown. One small portion is plenty. Make for dinner, or this is great to freeze for reheating.

Serves four.

STUFFED PASTA SHELL SALAD

8 jumbo pasta shells, cooked
2 tbsp. non-fat Italian dressing
⅔ cup cottage cheese
½ cup part-skim ricotta cheese

2 tbsp. minced scallions
1 tsp. lemon juice
⅛ tsp. grated lemon peel
Dash salt and freshly ground black pepper

In a shallow glass or stainless-steel bowl, combine boiled shells and dressing; toss to coat. Cover with plastic wrap and let marinate in refrigerator until chilled. In a small bowl combine remaining ingredients. Using a slotted spoon, remove shells from bowl, without dressing. Spoon cheese mixture into each shell; set shells on serving platter and drizzle with reserved dressing.

Serves two.

Easy Tuna Salad

2 cups romaine lettuce
1 cup finely chopped broccoli
1 cup halved grapes
1 tomato, chopped
1 6-oz. can tuna, drained and flaked
½ cup mandarin oranges, drained
2 tsp. low-fat mayonnaise
2 tsp. cider vinegar
⅛ tsp. freshly ground black pepper

Combine all ingredients and toss. This is a great afternoon treat.

Serves one.

Summer Salad

Dash salt and freshly ground black pepper
½ cucumber, sliced
2 medium oranges, peeled and cut

½ cup chopped green pepper
2 tbsp. chopped fresh parsley
½ cup plain low-fat yogurt
¼ tsp. dried thyme
2 cups romaine or any dark lettuce

In a mixing bowl, combine salt and pepper with cucumber, then toss with oranges, green pepper, and parsley. Combine yogurt and thyme in a separate bowl and mix, then add to first mixture and toss. Tear lettuce into separate serving bowl and add a small portion of mixture to taste. Top with freshly ground black pepper.

Serves one or two.

RICE AND ARTICHOKES

½ cup uncooked instant rice
½ 8-oz. can stewed tomatoes
½ 6-oz. can artichoke hearts
1 small green onion, chopped
½ tsp. salt

In a 10-inch skillet, mix all ingredients and bring to a boil. Stir frequently, reducing heat to low. Simmer, covered, for about 10 minutes, until rice is tender.

Serves two.

RICE WITH HERBS

3 tbsp. unsalted butter
1 cup uncooked brown rice
1 cup chopped yellow onion
2 cups water
3 tsp. chicken-broth granules

½ tsp. marjoram
½ tsp. salt
½ tsp. savory
½ cup almonds
1 tbsp. honey

In a medium saucepan on medium-high heat melt butter, adding rice and onion, and cook until lightly golden, 4 to 6 minutes. Add remaining ingredients, except almonds and honey, and bring to a boil, stirring occasionally. Cover the pan, lower the heat, and cook 15 to 20 minutes, until rice is tender. In the meantime, put almonds in a shallow pan, drizzle honey over them and place under broiler for about 5 minutes to toast. When rice is done, remove to serving plate(s) and top with almonds. A nice side dish for dinner, or a good light afternoon meal.

Serves four.

Rice and Vegetable Stir-Fry

¼ cup fat-free low-salt chicken broth
1 tbsp. olive oil
1 medium yellow onion, chopped
2 tsp. minced garlic
2 cups sliced frozen bell peppers
2 cups cooked wild rice
¼ cup fresh chopped parsley
¼ cup low-salt soy sauce

Heat broth and oil in a 10-inch skillet on medium-high heat. Add onion and garlic and cook about 8 minutes, stirring frequently, until onion is tender. Add peppers and rice. Stir-fry for approximately 2 minutes. Add parsley and soy sauce, and heat through. Great for a light lunch at home or office.

Serves two.

EVENING DISHES

The following are dishes that include appetizers, soups, special salads, side dishes, and main dishes. I want to emphasize that I don't choose a dish from each category for my meal. In fact I may have just two, and many times I have only one. Just a soup or salad or a brown rice dish, for example, can be satisfying as well as smart and healthy.

Most cooking time is spent on evening dishes. This is probably the time you cook for your family if you have one. Whether cooking for others or just for myself, I work by the same philosophy: Keep it smart and simple. Remember, do not eat too late in the evening, as most active, calorie-burning activities are done during the morning and afternoon. This is why I recommend some sort of evening exercise, like a walk, to keep your metabolism operating efficiently for optimum calorie burning. At my house we try to have a family activity after dinner. I try not to eat after 9 P.M. You've probably heard not to eat after 7 P.M., but my schedule runs late, and I allow for that. Eat to live, don't live to eat!

STUFFED MUSHROOMS

1 cup fresh spinach
10–12 medium-size mushrooms
1 tbsp. unsalted butter
1 clove garlic, minced
¼ tsp. oregano
1 tbsp. lemon juice
2 eggs
2 tbsp. bread crumbs

Preheat oven to 400°. Use a medium-size baking pan sprayed with non-stick spray. Place spinach (damp) in saucepan and cook over medium heat for 2 minutes. Put in strainer, squeezing out moisture, then chop. Remove stems from mushrooms and finely chop just the stems. In a small skillet heat butter, then cook garlic for a minute. Add chopped mushroom stems, then spinach and oregano, cooking for a few minutes. Stir in lemon juice, then remove from heat. In a small bowl beat eggs. Place bread crumbs in a small bowl. Take mushroom caps, dip in egg one at a time, and coat with bread crumbs. Fill each mushroom cap with spinach mixture and place in pan. Bake uncovered for 12 minutes until lightly browned. Great as an appetizer or served as a side dish.

Serves four.

Veggie-Stuffed Mushrooms

10–12 large mushrooms
1 tbsp. unsalted butter
1 tbsp. minced garlic
5 scallions, chopped
1 celery stalk, chopped
2 Roma tomatoes, cored and chopped
1 tbsp. chopped fresh basil
1 tbsp. chopped fresh parsley
1 tsp. freshly ground black pepper
2 eggs
½ cup bread crumbs
2 tbsp. grated Parmesan cheese

Preheat oven to 400°. Break off mushroom stems and chop fine. In a large skillet, melt butter on medium heat, adding garlic, scallions, celery, and chopped stems, and cook for 3 to 5 minutes. Add tomatoes, basil, parsley, and pepper and cook 3 to 4 minutes longer. Take off heat. Beat eggs in a small bowl. Put bread crumbs and Parmesan in a small bowl and mix. Dip each mushroom cap in egg, coat with crumbs and cheese, then stuff with veggie mix and place on a pan sprayed with

non-stick spray. Bake 15 minutes or until golden brown. Serve. Great
as an appetizer or as a side dish with a filet mignon.

Serves four.

Mushroom Salad

½ cup fat-free sour cream
1½ tbsp. lemon juice
1 clove garlic, minced
1 tsp. dried dill weed
½ tsp. salt
¼ tsp. freshly ground black pepper
1 8-oz. pkg. sliced mushrooms
3 large tomatoes, chopped

In a large bowl, whisk together sour cream, lemon juice, garlic, dill
weed, salt, and pepper until smooth and combined. Stir in mushrooms and tomatoes. Cover and refrigerate until ready to serve. Serve
as a side dish.

Serves four.

Stuffed Peppers

4 large green peppers
1 16-oz. pkg. frozen corn
1 cup boiling water
Dash salt and freshly ground black pepper
1 cup shelled baby lima beans, cooked and drained
1 large tomato, chopped
¼ cup chopped onion
½ tsp. dried rosemary, crushed
2 tbsp. melted unsalted butter

Cut peppers in half, and core. Cook peppers in boiling, lightly salted water for 3 to 5 minutes; drain. Measure 1½ cups corn. In a covered pan cook corn in 1 cup of boiling water 12 to 15 minutes or until done; drain the corn. Season green peppers with salt and pepper. Toss lima beans, tomato, onion, and rosemary together. Add cooked corn. Fill peppers with vegetable mixture. Spread butter at bottom of a medium-size baking dish and lay peppers in dish. Bake in a 350° oven for 30 minutes and serve.

Serves four.

SPINACH BALLS
Grandma Craig's Specialty

1 tbsp. unsalted butter
2 yellow onions, chopped
1½ cups fresh chopped spinach
4 cloves garlic, minced
1 tbsp. bread crumbs
1 tsp. grated lemon rind
1 tbsp. grated Parmesan cheese
½ tsp. freshly ground black pepper
1 egg white
1 8-oz. can tomato sauce
½ cup low-salt chicken broth
½ tsp. dried basil

Melt half the butter in a skillet on medium heat. Add half the onion and cook for 3 to 5 minutes. Add spinach and 2 tablespoons of garlic and cook, covered, for another 4 or 5 minutes. Preheat oven to 350°. Remove skillet from heat and stir in bread crumbs, lemon rind, Parmesan, half the black pepper, and the egg white. Put into a large bowl, mixing if needed. Shape contents into 1½-inch balls. Refrigerate. In a small saucepan, melt remaining butter over medium heat, adding remaining onion, cooking for 3 to 5 minutes. Add remaining garlic

(2 tablespoons) and pepper and tomato sauce, broth, and basil. Cover and simmer for about 20 minutes. In the meantime, place spinach balls in a baking pan sprayed with non-stick spray. Bake for about 30 minutes. Place balls in a serving dish and coat with tomato sauce. Serve.

These are a healthy appetizer when having company for dinner, and they are great cold or reheated as an afternoon snack.

Serves four.

CREAMY CUCUMBERS

1 small cucumber, peeled and sliced
½ red onion, sliced thin and separated into rings
¼ cup plain fat-free yogurt
½ tsp. chopped dill
⅛ tsp. freshly ground black pepper

Mix all ingredients and refrigerate, covered, for 4 hours. Makes a good side dish or salad course.

Serves one.

MARINATED VEGETABLES

½ cup white wine vinegar
1 tbsp. olive oil
1 clove garlic, sliced thin
½ tsp. paprika
1 tsp. freshly ground black pepper
1 cup water
2 medium carrots, thinly cut lengthwise
1 zucchini, thinly cut lengthwise
1 sweet red pepper, cored and thinly cut lengthwise
1 celery stalk, thinly cut lengthwise
1 tbsp. capers

In a medium-size pan, mix vinegar, oil, garlic, paprika, black pepper, and water. Add vegetables and capers, toss, cover, and refrigerate. This is great to serve on a salad plate with meat or seafood.

Serves four.

PARMESAN VEGGIES

1 cup sliced carrots
Dash salt
1 cup cauliflower, broken apart
1 green pepper, cored and sliced
2 tbsp. grated Parmesan cheese
1 tbsp. chopped fresh parsley
2 tbsp. butter
1 tsp. ground nutmeg

Put carrots in a steam basket and sprinkle with a little salt. Steam carrots for 5 minutes. Add cauliflower and steam 6 more minutes. Add green pepper and steam 3 more minutes. In a small bowl, mix grated Parmesan and chopped parsley. Toward the end of steaming, melt butter in a small saucepan, stirring in nutmeg. Take out veggies, put them in a bowl, and add butter mixture. Sprinkle with Parmesan mix and toss. This is another great side dish, and it's delicious for lunch by itself.

Serves six.

GARDENBURGER FIRE-ROASTED FOCACCIA

4 Gardenburger Fire-Roasted Vegetable patties
1 loaf focaccia bread, halved horizontally
2 tbsp. pesto sauce
4 roasted red peppers
4 thin slices yellow onion
½ cup shredded low-fat mozzarella cheese
Dash freshly ground black pepper

Toast or heat Gardenburger patties in a non-stick skillet until crisp and thoroughly heated. Spread bottom half of bread with pesto sauce. Layer red peppers, Gardenburger patties, and onion on pesto. Sprinkle cheese and pepper on cut side of top half of bread. Bake both halves at 375° for 10 minutes or until cheese melts. Place top half of bread, cut side down, on onion. Cut into 4 wedges. Great with a salad.

Serves four.

PARMESAN TOMATOES

2 tbsp. minced parsley
1 clove garlic, minced
¼ tsp. freshly ground black pepper
1 tsp. olive oil
4 large ripe tomatoes, cored and sliced thick
2½ tbsp. grated Parmesan cheese

Preheat broiler. In a small bowl mix parsley, garlic, and pepper. Coat a flat baking dish with oil. Arrange tomato slices in dish and sprinkle with parsley mixture, then cheese. Broil for about 3 minutes on top rack, being careful not to overcook. Great as a side dish.

Serves four.

BROWN RICE WITH ASPARAGUS

1 cup uncooked brown rice
1 egg and 1 egg white
1 tbsp. water
¼ tsp. sugar
2 tsp. low-salt soy sauce
⅓ lb. asparagus, cut
1 6-oz. pkg. frozen snow peas
1 tbsp. corn oil

4 cloves garlic, minced
1 tbsp. minced ginger
2 green onions, sliced
1 sweet red pepper, chopped
1 carrot, grated
6 cashews, roasted
2 tsp. white wine vinegar

Prepare rice according to directions, then put in the freezer to cool. In the meantime, beat the eggs with water, sugar, and a splash of the soy sauce: Cook like an omelette in a small non-stick pan on medium heat for 2 to 3 minutes. Take eggs out of pan (should be flat—a half moon) and cut into strips. In a separate saucepan, cook asparagus and snow peas in boiling water for about 30 seconds. Put in a strainer and rinse with cold water. Heat oil in a large skillet (or wok) on medium high and add garlic and ginger, stirring for a minute. Then add egg strips, asparagus, snow peas, onions, red pepper, carrot, cashews, and cooked rice, and cook, stirring, for 2 minutes. Mix in soy sauce and vinegar, then stir a minute. Serve.

Serves two.

GLAZED CARROTS

1 tbsp. unsalted butter
¾ cup orange juice
1½ tbsp. minced fresh ginger
8 carrots, sliced ¼ inch thick
Dried parsley (for garnish)

Melt butter in medium-size saucepan, then add orange juice and ginger. Bring to a boil. Add carrots and simmer for about 10 minutes. Garnish with parsley and serve.

Serves two or three.

MARINATED PEPPERS

2 each small sweet red, green, and yellow peppers
1 tbsp. olive oil
1 tbsp. red wine vinegar
1 clove garlic, minced
½ tsp. dried oregano
½ tsp. freshly ground black pepper

Put whole peppers on a flat pan and broil for about 5 minutes, turning 3 or 4 times until slightly darkened. Set aside to cool. Then remove the stems and core each, saving the juices in a large bowl. Cut peppers into small strips. Add all other ingredients to the bowl with the juices. Mix. Place peppers in bowl, mixing around. Cover and let sit for an hour before serving.

Peppers are something I like to eat frequently. These are great as a light lunch with a small broiled chicken breast.

Serves two.

SAUTÉED PEPPERS

1 tbsp. olive oil
2 sweet red peppers, cored and cut into small pieces
1 green pepper, cored and cut into small pieces
1 yellow onion, cut into large pieces
2 medium-size ripe tomatoes, cored and chopped
2 tbsp. cider vinegar
2 cloves garlic, minced

In a large skillet, heat oil on medium heat for a minute, then add peppers and onion. Lower heat slightly and cover, cooking for 7 to 10 minutes. Stir in tomatoes, vinegar, and garlic, cover, and cook 7 to 10 minutes more. Serve. These are a great side dish.

Serves two.

ZUCCHINI CASSEROLE

1 tsp. olive oil
3 zucchini, sliced thin
1 large white onion, chopped
1 ripe tomato, chopped
Dash salt and freshly ground black pepper
3 eggs and 3 egg whites
Dash garlic powder
1 tbsp. oregano
⅓ cup grated **Parmesan cheese**

Preheat oven to 350°. In a medium skillet heat oil on medium-high heat and sauté zucchini and onion for a minute, adding tomato, salt, and pepper. Continue to sauté until onion is slightly brown. In a large bowl, beat eggs and mix in garlic powder and oregano. Add zucchini mixture and mix in cheese. Bake in casserole dish for 45 minutes and serve.

Serves three.

ZUCCHINI IN TOMATO SAUCE

¼ cup unsalted butter
2 lbs. zucchini, sliced into ½-inch pieces
½ cup chopped onion
1 14-oz. can tomato sauce
1 carrot, grated
1 tsp. salt
½ tsp. (fresh or dried) basil
½ tsp. (fresh or dried) oregano
¼ tsp. freshly ground black pepper
¼ tsp. garlic powder
½ cup grated Romano cheese

In a large skillet on medium heat, melt butter and brown zucchini and onion lightly. In a bowl combine all other ingredients except cheese. Add mixture to the skillet and simmer for 15 minutes, until zucchini is tender. Take off the heat and put on a serving dish. Top with Romano and serve.

Serves four.

ZUCCHINI PARMESAN

1½ cups zucchini, cut lengthwise into strips
6 garlic cloves
½ cup bread crumbs
¼ cup grated Parmesan cheese
1 cup non-fat milk
1 egg
⅛ tsp. ground nutmeg
¼ tsp. salt
¼ tsp. freshly ground black pepper
½ cup fat-free ricotta cheese
1 cup chopped cherry tomatoes
¼ cup chopped fresh basil
1 tsp. olive oil

Preheat broiler. Place zucchini and garlic on a baking sheet that is sprayed with non-stick spray. Broil about 5 minutes until lightly browned. Take garlic out and mince, and set zucchini aside. Preheat oven to 400°. Combine garlic, bread crumbs, and Parmesan in a small bowl. Combine milk, egg, nutmeg, salt, pepper, and ricotta in a medium bowl and mix well. In a separate bowl, mix tomatoes, basil, and oil. Spread ½ cup of the milk mixture on the bottom of a baking dish coated with non-stick spray. Arrange zucchini slices over milk mixture to cover the bottom, and top with one-third of the bread-crumb mix, then another ½ cup milk mixture, repeating until zucchini is on top. Top with tomato mix and sprinkle with remaining bread-crumb mix. Bake for about 40 minutes until slightly brown. This is a great side dish.

Serves six.

ITALIAN ZUCCHINI BOWLS

2 large zucchini, halved lengthwise
1 tbsp. unsalted butter
1 tsp. minced garlic
¼ cup chopped onion
½ cup chopped green pepper
½ cup chopped tomato
½ tsp. dried basil
½ cup low-fat cottage cheese
1 tbsp. grated Parmesan cheese

Preheat oven to 350°. With a spoon, scoop out centers of halved zucchini, forming a shell. Chop scooped-out portion. In a medium skillet, melt butter on medium heat and add garlic and onion, then pepper, tomato, basil, and chopped zucchini—sauté for 3 or 4 minutes. Stir in cottage cheese. Take off heat and spoon into shells. Bake 15 minutes. Top with Parmesan and serve.

Serves three or four.

BRUSSELS SPROUTS WITH ALMONDS

1 lb. brussels sprouts
2 tbsp. unsalted butter
1 cup chopped almonds
2 tbsp. lemon juice

Simmer sprouts in a medium skillet until tender. Put in a serving bowl. In a small skillet on medium heat, melt butter, then add almonds and lemon juice, cooking until almonds are brown. Pour mixture onto sprouts and toss. Serve.

Serves four.

BROCCOLI SIDE

2 heads broccoli
2 tbsp. unsalted butter
1 tsp. minced garlic
½ tsp. basil
2 tbsp. lemon juice

Cut stems off broccoli, wash, and steam for about 12 minutes. Place in strainer. In a small skillet on medium heat, melt butter, then add garlic and cook for a minute. Add basil and lemon juice and simmer a minute. Put broccoli in a serving dish, toss with garlic mix, and serve.

Serves four.

ASPARAGUS WITH SESAME SEEDS

1 cup cut-up asparagus, hard parts of stems removed
1½ tsp. unsalted butter
1 tbsp. sesame seeds
1 tsp. low-salt soy sauce
1 tsp. sesame oil
½ tsp. freshly ground black pepper

Steam asparagus for about 5 minutes. Drain and rinse with cold water. In a large saucepan, melt butter and add sesame seeds; cook for 3 minutes on medium-high heat. Add asparagus, soy sauce, sesame oil, and pepper and cook for a minute or two.

Serves one.

GREEN BEANS AND DILL

1½ cups trimmed fresh green beans
1½ tsp. unsalted butter
2 tsp. lemon juice
½ tsp. freshly ground black pepper
2 tbsp. snipped fresh dill

Steam green beans for about 6 minutes. Drain and rinse with cold water. In a large saucepan, melt butter on medium heat. Put green beans in saucepan and cook for about 2 minutes. Add lemon juice, pepper, and dill. Mix thoroughly and serve. This is a delicious side dish.

Serves one.

HERB-GRILLED VEGETABLES

2 tbsp. minced garlic
2 tbsp. olive oil
1 tsp. freshly ground black pepper
1 tsp. (fresh or dried) oregano
1 tsp. (fresh or dried) rosemary
1 tsp. (fresh or dried) thyme
1 carrot, sliced into ½-inch pieces
1 red bell pepper, thickly sliced
1 yellow squash, halved and sliced
1 zucchini, halved and sliced

In a large bowl, combine all ingredients except vegetables and mix. Add vegetables and toss to coat evenly. Heat a medium-large non-stick pan on medium heat and add vegetables and cook, stirring often, until tender and slightly charred in spots (about 5 minutes). Serve immediately with tuna steaks or with another main dish.

This is great with brown rice. You can also make it the night before and reheat it for lunch.

Serves four.

Spinach Casserole

1 egg and 2 egg whites
3 tbsp. flour
1 10-oz. pkg. frozen chopped spinach, thawed
12 oz. cottage cheese
1 tsp. freshly ground black pepper
Dash salt
8 oz. sliced low-fat Lorraine Swiss cheese

Preheat oven to 350°. In a large bowl, beat eggs, add flour, and mix thoroughly until smooth. Add spinach, cottage cheese, pepper, and salt and mix well. Pour half of the mixture into a non-stick-sprayed baking pan, layer Lorraine Swiss slices evenly on top, and pour remaining mixture over all. Bake uncovered for 1 hour. Let stand to cool a bit, then serve. Good to serve with meat.

Serves four.

Baked Asparagus

2 tsp. unsalted butter
1 cup asparagus, hard parts of stems removed
2½ tbsp. grated Parmesan cheese
1½ tbsp. bread crumbs

Preheat oven to 400°. Melt butter in a small microwave-safe bowl. Spread evenly in medium-size baking pan. Then place asparagus in a single layer in baking pan. Sprinkle on Parmesan and bread crumbs. Bake for about 10 minutes, uncovered, and serve.

Serves one.

ASPARAGUS WITH LEMON VINAIGRETTE

1 lb. fresh asparagus (or broccoli)
¼ cup fresh lemon juice
2 tsp. olive oil
½ tsp. salt
¼ tsp. freshly ground black pepper
Parsley or basil (for garnish)

Steam asparagus until tender, either in a microwave-safe dish with ½ cup or more of water, covered, or in a steamer above boiling water, covered, until tender, about 6 minutes. In a small bowl, mix lemon juice, oil, salt, and pepper. Put asparagus in a bowl, and add lemon mix. Or place individual servings on plates and pour a moderate amount of sauce over them. Garnish with parsley or basil. Serve as a side dish with fish.

Serves three or four.

ROASTED POTATOES

½ lb. halved tiny red potatoes
3 garlic cloves
1 tsp. olive oil
Dash freshly ground black pepper
1 tbsp. chives

Preheat oven to 350°. In an ovenproof casserole dish, arrange potatoes in a single layer. Put garlic cloves among the potatoes. Drizzle on olive oil and sprinkle pepper. Bake 30 to 40 minutes until tender and garlic is soft. Squeeze garlic cloves onto potatoes. Sprinkle with pepper and chives. This is a nice accompaniment to a beef or chicken dish.

Serves three or four.

Peppy Potatoes

2 large potatoes, peeled and thinly sliced
2 tbsp. olive oil
6 sweet cherry tomatoes, sliced
½ cup sliced yellow onion
½ cup grated Romano cheese
¼ cup sliced mushrooms
Dash salt and freshly ground black pepper

In a large skillet brown potatoes in oil on medium heat for about 20 minutes. Add all other ingredients, including salt and pepper, and simmer for about 10 minutes. Serve. Good as a side dish with meat.

Serves four.

Mushroom Soup

½ cup pearl barley
1½ cups water
4 cups low-salt beef broth
2 tsp. olive oil
1 clove garlic, minced
1 small yellow onion, chopped
2 small celery stalks, finely chopped
¼ lb. leanest ground round
¼ lb. fresh mushrooms
½ tsp. Worcestershire sauce
⅛ tsp. (fresh or dried) thyme
⅛ tsp. (fresh or dried) marjoram
Dash salt
¼ tsp. freshly ground black pepper

Place barley in a bowl with water and soak overnight. The next day, bring broth to a light boil in a medium pot, add the water with barley, and cook, uncovered, about 45 minutes until tender. In the mean-time, heat oil in a non-stick skillet. Add garlic and onion and sauté for 5 or 6 minutes. Add celery and sauté 3 or 4 minutes. Add ground round and sauté another 4 or 5 minutes, then add mushrooms and cook for another 4 minutes. To the tender barley add Worcestershire, thyme, marjoram, salt, and pepper. Stir in the sautéed mixture and serve.

Serves four.

VEGETABLE AND TORTELLINI SOUP

¼ cup water
½ cup peas
½ cup carrots, cut lengthwise into 1-inch strips
6 oz. tortellini (meat or cheese)
4 cups low-salt chicken broth
1 8-oz. can mushrooms, drained
2 tbsp. freshly grated Parmesan cheese

In a microwave-safe dish, combine water with peas and carrots and cook, covered, on high for 2 minutes until steamed thoroughly and tender. Cook tortellini according to directions, until al dente. In a medium pot, bring broth to a light boil. Add peas, carrots, mushrooms, and tortellini. Ladle into serving bowls. Sprinkle with Parmesan.

Serves six to eight.

SEAFOOD GAZPACHO

1 12- or 14-oz. can Italian plum tomatoes, diced
½ cup low-salt beef broth
¼ cup peeled and chopped cucumber
¼ cup chopped green pepper
¼ cup chopped white onion

2 cloves garlic, minced
1 tbsp. olive oil
1½ tsp. fresh lemon juice
Dash each ground cumin, Tabasco, salt, (fresh or dried) basil
8 oz. cooked shrimp meat

In a medium-large bowl, combine all ingredients except shrimp and chill for at least 2 hours. Add shrimp before serving. This is a nice light evening meal with a slice of bread. Or it makes an easy lunch.

Serves two to four.

SEAFOOD GUMBO

2 tbsp. unsalted butter
2 medium-size yellow onions, minced
1 clove garlic, minced
1 small sweet green pepper, chopped
1 medium-size celery stalk, chopped
4 tsp. flour
3 cups low-salt chicken broth
1 14-oz. can low-salt chopped tomatoes
½ cup chopped low-salt ham
1 large bay leaf
¼ tsp. hot pepper sauce
1 cup uncooked enriched long-grain rice
1 10-oz. pkg. frozen okra
½ lb. medium shrimp, deveined
1 10-oz. can crabmeat
1 10-oz. jar oysters

In a large saucepan, melt butter over medium heat. Add onions and garlic and sauté for 4 minutes. Mix in green pepper and celery, and cook, stirring frequently, for another 4 minutes. Add flour and cook for a minute. Stir in broth, tomatoes with juice, ham, bay leaf, and pepper sauce. Simmer, partially covered, for about 30 minutes. (At this point prepare rice according to instructions on package.) Add okra and continue cooking another 30 minutes. Add shrimp and crabmeat the last 5 minutes of simmering, and stir in oysters the last 2 minutes. Spoon gumbo onto rice and serve.

Serves four.

CRAB CHOWDER

1 large yellow onion, chopped
1 potato, peeled and chopped
1 celery stalk, sliced thin
1 carrot, peeled and sliced thin
½ tsp. dried thyme
½ tsp. dried basil
1½ cups water
1 cup skim milk
2 tbsp. flour
⅛ tsp. cayenne pepper
1 8-oz. can crabmeat
2 tbsp. chopped parsley

In a medium-size saucepan, combine onion, potato, celery, carrot, thyme, basil, and water. Cook over medium heat until mixture bubbles gently, then simmer, uncovered, for 15 minutes. In a small bowl, blend milk, flour, and cayenne pepper until smooth. Stir into vegetable mixture, then return to a simmer, stirring constantly, and cook 3 minutes longer. Add crabmeat and cook another 5 minutes. Sprinkle each serving with parsley.

Serves two.

Roast Sirloin

2 tbsp. black peppercorns
1 lb. boneless lean sirloin, fat trimmed
1 tbsp. olive oil
4 scallions, chopped
2 tbsp. white cooking wine
1 cup low-salt beef broth

Crush peppercorns and coat sirloin with them. Put oil in an ovenproof skillet and set on high. After about a minute add sirloin and sear for about 30 seconds on each side. Then put the skillet in a preheated 550° oven, uncovered, and cook for 5 or 6 minutes. Take out steak and slice thinly. Put scallions in skillet and cook on medium heat for half a minute, adding wine, then broth a minute later. Simmer for 2 minutes. Serve with the drippings. Roast sirloin is delicious served with steamed carrots.

Serves two.

Beef Tenderloin

½ cup low-salt chicken broth
2 large onions, thinly sliced
4 cloves garlic, finely chopped
¼ cup balsamic vinegar
1 tsp. olive oil
½ tsp. salt
¼ tsp. freshly ground black pepper
4 beef tenderloin steaks, about 1 inch thick (1 lb. total)

Heat ¼ cup broth to boiling in a 1-quart saucepan. Stir in onions and garlic; reduce heat to medium. Cover and cook about 15 minutes, stirring occasionally, until onions are soft and brown, adding remaining broth to prevent onions from sticking. Stir in vinegar. Cook, uncovered, on medium-high heat about 2 minutes until liquid has evaporated; remove from heat. During that time heat medium non-stick skillet on medium-high heat and add oil. Sprinkle salt and pepper on beef and cook it in the skillet for about 8 minutes for medium doneness, turning once. Add onion mix and serve.

Serves four.

BEEF TENDERLOIN DELIGHT

½ cup fat-free low-salt chicken broth
2 large yellow onions, minced
4 tbsp. minced garlic
¼ cup balsamic vinegar
1 tsp. olive oil
4 beef tenderloin steaks, about 1 inch thick (1 lb. total)
½ tsp. salt
1 tbsp. freshly ground black pepper

In a 1-quart saucepan, bring broth to a light boil and stir in onions and garlic. Reduce heat to medium and cover, cooking for about 15 minutes and stirring occasionally until onions are soft and light brown. Stir in vinegar and, after 2 more minutes when most of liquid has evaporated, take off heat. Spread oil in a skillet and heat on medium high. Put in beef and cook for about 8 minutes, sprinkling half of salt and pepper on one side, turning beef halfway through, and adding remaining salt and pepper. Take off heat, place on serving dish, pour sauce on top, and serve.

Serves four.

ELEGANT LINGUINE WITH ASPARAGUS VINAIGRETTE

1½ tbsp. dark sesame oil
1 tbsp. peeled minced fresh ginger
¼ tsp. crushed red pepper

3 cloves garlic, minced
1½ cups sliced shiitake mushroom caps
1 cup sliced button mushrooms
¼ cup rice vinegar
2 tbsp. low-salt soy sauce
¼ cup minced fresh parsley
¼ cup pineapple juice
2 tbsp. water
2 tsp. sugar
1 lb. asparagus spears
8 oz. cooked linguine

Heat oil in a large non-stick skillet. Add ginger, pepper, and garlic; cook 1 minute. Add mushrooms; cook 2 minutes. Add vinegar, soy sauce, parsley, pineapple juice, water, and sugar; remove from heat. Snap off tough ends of asparagus and remove scales with a knife or vegetable peeler, if desired. Brush asparagus with mushroom vinaigrette (keep remaining vinaigrette). Roast asparagus at 450° for 10 minutes or until tender. Place cooked asparagus over pasta. Pour remaining vinaigrette over asparagus and serve.

Serves two or three.

Pineapple Pork Chops

3 tbsp. minced garlic
½ cup canned pineapple cubes with juice
1 tbsp. honey mustard
4 lean pork chops, trimmed
2 tbsp. Italian bread crumbs (optional)
¼ tsp. salt
¼ tsp. freshly ground black pepper

Shake garlic, pineapple, and honey mustard in a sealable plastic bag. Put in pork chops (fat trimmed) and shake again. You can put this in the refrigerator and let marinate for 1 hour, or put bread crumbs in bag and shake well again. Cook the drained chops in a skillet on medium-high heat for about 3 minutes per side. Sprinkle with salt and pepper and add marinade from bag when a minute or two from being done. Turn heat to low and simmer about 5 minutes, then serve.

Serves four.

PORK WITH BASIL

¾ lb. lean pork tenderloin
1 tsp. vegetable oil
¼ cup chopped fresh basil leaves
¼ cup low-salt chicken broth
4 cloves garlic, chopped
⅛ tsp. cayenne pepper

Trim fat from pork. Cut pork crosswise into 8 pieces. Flatten each piece to ¼-inch thickness. Heat oil in medium non-stick skillet over medium-high heat. Cook pork in oil about 4 minutes, turning once, until brown. Stir in remaining ingredients. Heat to boil, reduce heat to low. Cover and simmer about 5 minutes or until pork is slightly pink in center. This is great served with fresh steamed greens.

Serves two or three.

GRILLED PORK CHOPS

4 loin pork chops, about ½ inch thick (2 lbs.)
1 clove garlic, chopped
1 tbsp. chili powder
1 tsp. ground cumin
¼ tsp. cayenne pepper
¼ tsp. salt

Trim fat from chops. In a small bowl, mix remaining ingredients. Rub chili-powder mixture evenly on both sides of chops. Cover and refrigerate 1 hour to blend flavors. Heat coals or gas grill for direct heat. Cover and grill chops 4 to 6 inches from heat, 10 to 12 minutes, turning frequently and brushing chops with mixture, until slightly pink when cut near bone.

Serves four.

PEPPER STEAK

2 tsp. olive oil
1½–2 lbs. thin sirloin, cut into strips
1 green pepper, cut into strips
1 large onion, sliced
1 celery stalk, chopped
1 tsp. seasoned salt
1 beef bouillon cube dissolved in 1 cup of water
¼ cup catsup
1 tbsp. cornstarch
¼ cup water
¼ cup soy sauce
1 cup sliced mushroom caps

In a large skillet on medium-high heat, heat oil and brown meat, green pepper, onion, and celery. Sprinkle with seasoned salt and cook 5 minutes. Then add beef bouillon and catsup and cook for 5 more minutes. Put cornstarch in water and mix thoroughly. Add to skillet slowly, while stirring. Add soy sauce and mushrooms. Cover and cook until meat is tender, about 30 minutes, and serve.

Serves four.

Steak with Brown Rice

½ cup uncooked brown rice
1 tbsp. olive oil
1 10-oz. beef tenderloin steaks, cut into ½-inch-thick strips
2 green onions, chopped
⅓ cup low-salt beef broth
1 tsp. grated lemon rind
¼ tsp. freshly ground black pepper
3 tbsp. minced parsley

Prepare rice according to directions. In the meantime, in a medium skillet heat oil over medium-high heat and add steak strips. Cook until the outside is no longer pink, 2 or 3 minutes (or until slightly *underdone*, to your taste). Put meat aside on a plate. Add green onions, beef broth, lemon rind, and pepper to the skillet. Cook 4 to 6 minutes, until half the liquid is evaporated. Put meat back in, along with parsley, and toss, heating through. This should cook the meat to your taste. Serve over rice.

Serves two.

Lemon Chicken

½ cup low-salt chicken broth
2 skinless, boneless chicken breasts
2 tbsp. olive oil
¼ cup flour
3 tbsp. lemon juice
½ tsp. paprika
½ cup sliced mushrooms
2 tbsp. capers

Heat a medium-size skillet and bring broth to a light boil. Meanwhile, cut chicken in half, pounding to half its thickness. Brush with oil. Broil for 3 to 5 minutes on each side. Set chicken aside on serving plate. Add flour a little at a time to broth and turn heat to low, stirring frequently until sauce thickens. Then add lemon juice, paprika, mushrooms, and capers and simmer for a minute. Pour mixture over chicken and serve. Lemon Chicken is great served with steamed carrots or green beans.

Serves two.

CHICKEN BREASTS WITH PESTO

⅓ cup olive oil
3 medium-size summer squash, cut into 1-inch cubes
3 medium-size yellow bell peppers, cut into 1-inch squares
3 medium-size zucchini, cut into 1-inch slices
Dash salt and freshly ground black pepper
2 tbsp. fresh lemon juice
¼ cup pesto sauce
4 skinless, boneless chicken breasts, pounded to an even
    thickness

Preheat oven to 425°. In a large roasting pan set over 2 burners, heat oil. Add vegetables, season lightly with salt and pepper, and stir to coat with oil. Roast vegetables for 25 minutes or until tender. Transfer vegetables to a bowl and let cool. Stir in lemon juice and pesto. Preheat a grill pan. Rub chicken breasts with oil and season with salt and pepper. Grill chicken over high heat until lightly charred and just cooked through, about 4 minutes per side. Serve hot, topped with warmed pesto and vegetable mixture.

Serves four.

ORANGE CHICKEN

1 cup frozen orange juice concentrate, thawed
1 tsp. minced fresh oregano (or 1 tsp. dried)

Dash freshly ground black pepper
4 medium skinless, boneless chicken breasts

In a large non-stick skillet combine thawed concentrate, oregano, and pepper, and heat on medium. Place chicken in skillet. Bring to a boil; reduce heat. Cover and simmer for 10 minutes. Remove chicken, reserving juice mixture. Place chicken on the unheated rack of a broiler pan lined with foil. Broil 4 inches from heat for 2 minutes. Turn and brush with reserved juice mixture. Broil 2 minutes more until golden and no pink remains, then serve.

Serves four.

VEGETABLE-BEEF SOUP

15 oz. stew beef, cubed
1½ qts. water
¾ cup vegetable juice
½ cup chopped scallions
1½ oz. uncooked rinsed lentils
¼ cup chopped celery
¼ cup chopped green cabbage
¼ cup diced parsnips
¼ cup diced turnips
½ clove garlic, minced
1 tbsp. chopped basil
¾ tsp. salt
⅛ tsp. freshly ground black pepper
½ cup sliced mushrooms

In broiling pan broil beef, turning once, until rare and browned, about 5 minutes on each side. Transfer beef to 4-quart pot; add remaining ingredients except mushrooms and bring liquid to a boil. Reduce heat to low, cover pan, and let simmer, stirring occasionally, until meat and vegetables are tender, 40 to 50 minutes. Add mushrooms and cook for 1 to 2 minutes longer.

Serves four.

CHICKEN PITAS

¼ tsp. salt
2 tsp. plus 3 tbsp. olive oil
½ tsp. freshly ground black pepper
4 medium skinless, boneless chicken breasts, halved
3 tbsp. lemon juice
3 tbsp. light mayonnaise
1 tbsp. Dijon mustard
1 tsp. anchovy paste
1 small clove garlic, minced
½ cup grated Parmesan cheese
4 pitas (6- to 7-inch diameter)
4 cups shredded romaine lettuce

Preheat broiler. In a medium bowl mix salt, 2 teaspoons oil, and ¼ teaspoon pepper. Add chicken and stir to coat. Place chicken on rack in broiling pan. Broil on top rack, about 6 minutes each side, until juices run clear when thickest part is pierced with tip of knife. Take out, let cool. Mix lemon juice, mayonnaise, mustard, anchovy paste, garlic, 3 tablespoons oil, and remaining pepper; stir in Parmesan cheese. Slit top third of each pita to form an opening. Thinly slice chicken and add with lettuce to dressing; toss well. Fill pita with salad and serve.

Serves four.

PINEAPPLE CHICKEN STIR-FRY

2 tbsp. pineapple juice
½ cup chicken broth
1 tbsp. low-salt soy sauce
4 chicken breasts, cut into 3-inch strips
1 tsp. vegetable oil
2 celery stalks, sliced

½ cup diced zucchini
½ cup canned pineapple chunks
½ cup sliced mushroom caps
¼ cup sliced scallions
⅛ tsp. garlic powder
1 tsp. cornstarch

In a small glass bowl combine pineapple juice, broth, and soy sauce. Add chicken, stirring to coat thoroughly. Cover with plastic wrap and refrigerate for 30 minutes. Remove chicken from marinade, reserve marinade, and pat chicken dry. In wok or medium skillet heat oil over high heat and add chicken and cook, stirring quickly and frequently until lightly browned, 2 to 3 minutes. Transfer chicken to plate and keep warm. To same pan add celery and zucchini, stir-fry for 1 to 2 minutes; add pineapple, mushrooms, scallions, and garlic powder and stir-fry for 1 minute longer. Dissolve cornstarch in reserved marinade and add to pan along with chicken; cook 2 to 3 minutes until thickened and serve.

Serves four.

Chicken Primavera

2 cups water
1 cup diced carrots
1 cup broccoli flowerets
1 cup tri-color rigatoni pasta
4 medium skinless, boneless chicken breasts, broiled and cubed
½ cup plain non-fat yogurt
¼ cup finely chopped scallions
2 tbsp. and 2 tsp. low-calorie mayonnaise
2 tbsp. grated Parmesan cheese
½ tsp. crushed dried basil
⅛ tsp. freshly ground black pepper

In a medium saucepan combine water, carrots, and broccoli. Cook, covered, 10 to 15 minutes or until tender-crisp, and drain. Cook pasta according to package directions; rinse and drain. In a large bowl combine pasta, carrots, and broccoli and toss. In a small bowl combine chicken, yogurt, scallions, mayonnaise, Parmesan, basil, and pepper; mix well. Add to pasta mixture. Toss gently to combine. Cover and refrigerate several hours before serving.

Serves four.

CHICKEN BREAST WITH KIWI

⅓ cup buttermilk
1 tbsp. Dijon mustard
1 cup chopped parsley
½ cup bread crumbs
4 skinless, boneless chicken breasts, halved
2 tbsp. olive oil
1 clove garlic, minced
¼ cup low-salt chicken broth
4 kiwi fruit, peeled and thinly sliced

Mix buttermilk with Dijon mustard. In a separate bowl mix parsley and bread crumbs. Dip the halved chicken breasts in buttermilk mix, then roll in bowl of bread-crumb mix to coat. Heat oil in a skillet on medium-high heat and add garlic, then coated chicken, and sauté for about 6 minutes until golden brown. Remove chicken, keeping warm. To the same pan add broth, stirring to scrape up chicken bits in pan. Add kiwi, and cook 1 or 2 minutes or until sauce thickens slightly. Pour sauce over chicken and serve immediately.

Serves four.

HONEY CHICKEN

½ cup honey
2 tbsp. lemon juice

2 tbsp. Dijon mustard
2 tbsp. low-salt chicken broth
½ tsp. grated lemon peel
4 skinless, boneless chicken breasts

Preheat grill or broiler. Mix all ingredients except chicken in a medium bowl. Brush chicken with some of the honey mixture, and broil or grill chicken until tender, about 6 minutes per side or less, turning once and brushing again. Be careful not to overcook. Put the rest of the mixture in the microwave for about 30 seconds on high. Pour over chicken breasts. Serve with brown rice or a side salad. Healthy and easy!

Serves four.

CHICKEN CREOLE

4 skinless, boneless chicken breasts, cut into 1-inch strips
2 tbsp. water
1 14-oz. can tomatoes, chopped
1 cup low-salt chili sauce
1½ cups chopped green pepper
½ cup chopped celery
¼ cup chopped onion
2 cloves garlic, minced
1 tsp. chopped fresh basil
1 tbsp. chopped fresh parsley
¼ tsp. crushed red pepper
¼ tsp. salt

Spray deep skillet with non-stick spray. Preheat pan over high heat. Cook chicken in hot skillet, adding water to help steam the chicken. Stir for 3 to 5 minutes, or until no longer pink. Reduce heat. Add tomatoes and their juice, chili sauce, green pepper, celery, onion, garlic, basil, parsley, red pepper, and salt. Bring to a boil; reduce heat and simmer, covered, for 10 minutes. Serve over rice or whole-wheat pasta.

Serves four.

BROCCOLI CHICKEN

2 8-oz. skinless, boneless chicken breasts, cut into ½-inch strips
1 tsp. salt
1 tsp. freshly ground black pepper
2 tbsp. unsalted butter
¼ cup chopped onion
1 10-oz. pkg. frozen cut broccoli, thawed
1 tsp. lemon juice
¼ tsp. crushed dried thyme
3 medium-size tomatoes, cut into wedges

Season chicken strips with ¼ tsp. salt and pepper. Melt butter in a skillet and cook chicken and onion quickly on medium high until chicken is just done. Stir in broccoli, lemon juice, thyme, and remaining salt and pepper, turn heat to low, and cook, covered, for 6 minutes. Add tomatoes. Cook, covered, 3 to 4 minutes more. Great served with a side of greens.

Serves two.

MEDITERRANEAN PITA

1 Gardenburger Classic Greek veggie patty
1 whole-wheat pita bread
¼ cup chopped romaine lettuce
½ cucumber, sliced thinly
3 tomato slices
2 thinly sliced red onion rings
2 tbsp. Cucumber Yogurt Dill Sauce (below)

Cucumber Yogurt Dill Sauce:
¼ cup plain non-fat yogurt
2 tbsp. chopped cucumber

2 tsp. chopped red onion
1 tsp. (fresh or dried) dill
⅛ tsp. freshly ground black pepper
Dash garlic powder, cumin powder, and salt

In a small bowl combine ingredients for dill sauce and set aside. Prepare Gardenburger patty as directed on package. Cut pita bread in half and stuff with chopped-up patty, greens, cucumber, tomato, and red onion. Top with Cucumber Yogurt Dill Sauce. Great for lunch or as an afternoon snack.

Serves one.

Shrimp Kabobs

½ pound medium shrimp, thawed and deveined
1 tsp. sugar
¼ cup lemon juice
1 tbsp. balsamic vinegar
4 tbs. chopped fresh garlic
1 large red bell pepper, cut into squares
1 yellow onion, peeled and cut in half
2 cups not-so-thinly-sliced zucchini
2 tsp. olive oil

In a container with a lid, mix shrimp with sugar, lemon juice, balsamic vinegar, and garlic. Cover with lid and refrigerate for 1 hour. Put shrimp on skewers, alternating with each vegetable. Brush all pieces on skewer with oil. Put on flat oven pan covered with foil and broil on top rack 2 or 3 minutes each side. With a side of mandarin oranges and a glass of iced tea, you'll have a healthy and elegant meal.

Serves four.

SCAMPI AND PASTA

6 oz. spinach fettuccine
1 tsp. olive oil
½ lb. uncooked, peeled, deveined shrimp (thawed if frozen)
2 cloves garlic, chopped
2 tbsp. thinly sliced green onion
2 tbsp. lemon juice
1 tbsp. chopped fresh basil leaves
1 tbsp. chopped fresh parsley
¼ tsp. salt

Cook fettuccine according to directions on package. While fettuccine is cooking, heat oil over medium heat in a skillet. Place shrimp, garlic, and onion in pan for a minute, then add remaining ingredients and cook for another 2 or 3 minutes, stirring frequently, until shrimp are pink and firm; remove from heat. Toss fettuccine with shrimp mixture and serve. Make the shrimp the larger part of this dish—eat a small portion.

Serves two.

ELEGANT STEAMED CLAMS

4 qts. fresh clams, in shell
8 cups water
¼ cup dry white wine
2 tbsp. soy sauce
2 tbsp. lemon juice

Wash clams thoroughly under cold water. Scrub with brush to remove grime. Add clams to a large pot of boiling water, cover, and turn heat to low. Steam until clams are barely open, stirring occasionally. Strain. Put clam broth, wine, soy sauce, and lemon juice in a small pot and heat thoroughly. Serve clams in a bowl, pouring liquid into a small separate bowl for dipping. You may want an additional bowl for the shells. Great with a salad.

Serves five or six.

GRILLED SALMON

1 cup plain non-fat yogurt
1 tbsp. light mayonnaise
¼ cup minced green onions
1 tbsp. minced dill weed
2 tsp. lime juice
1 tsp. hot pepper sauce
1 12- to 16-oz skinned salmon fillets (1 inch thick)
1 tbsp. olive oil

In a small glass bowl combine yogurt, mayonnaise, green onions, dill weed, lime juice, and hot pepper sauce. Cover and chill at least 1 hour. Cut salmon into 4 equal portions; brush with oil. Grill salmon over medium-hot coals 5 minutes on each side or until fish flakes easily with fork. (Can be broiled if a grill is not available.) Top with yogurt mixture and serve with side of greens.

Serves four.

TUNA AND PASTA

1 cup sliced mushrooms
½ cup sliced onions
1 tbsp. olive oil
1 cup diced tomatoes
1 12-oz. can albacore tuna, drained and flaked
¼ cup fat-free chicken stock
Pinch red pepper flakes
8 oz. uncooked fettuccine
2 tbsp. minced fresh basil
3 tbsp. grated Parmesan cheese

In a large non-stick pan over medium-high heat, sauté mushrooms and onions in the oil for 5 minutes or until tender. Add tomatoes, tuna, stock, and pepper flakes. Cover and simmer over low heat for

5 minutes. Meanwhile, cook fettuccine according to package directions. Drain and place in a large bowl. Add tuna mixture and basil;
toss well to combine. Sprinkle with Parmesan. Great in the evening
or reheated for a delightful afternoon snack.

Serves four.

Tuna with Tomato-Basil Topping

2 tbsp. olive oil
2 cloves garlic, minced
3 medium-size ripe tomatoes, chopped fine
¼ cup finely chopped basil
½ tsp. salt
½ tsp. freshly ground black pepper
1 lb. fresh tuna (about 1 inch thick)
1 bunch red leaf lettuce (or romaine)

If grilling, prepare coals; or preheat broiler. In a blender, combine oil,
garlic, tomatoes, basil, salt, and half of the pepper and blend until
smooth. Set aside. Grill tuna 3 or 4 minutes on medium heat of grill
on a piece of foil with an abundance of small holes made with a fork,
or broil about same time, until done (turning once). Place large pieces
of lettuce on plates, place tuna on top, and add a small portion of
tomato blend, sprinkling remaining pepper on top. Serve with a vegetable.

Serves four.

Tuna with Almonds and Rice

1 cup uncooked brown rice
3 tbsp. all-purpose flour
1 tsp. curry powder
¼ tsp. dry mustard

1 cup low-fat milk
10 oz. water-packed tuna (about 1½ 6-oz. cans), drained and
    flaked
1 15-oz. can sliced mushrooms, drained
¼ cup lemon juice
2 tsp. freshly ground black pepper
3 tbsp. almonds

Cook brown rice according to directions. In the meantime, in a
medium-size bowl combine flour, curry powder, and dry mustard. Using
a whisk, add milk slowly and beat until smooth. Put in a large saucepan
and bring to a boil over medium-high heat, stirring constantly. Stir in
tuna, mushrooms, lemon juice, and pepper. Cook for another 1 or 2 minutes, stirring frequently. Toast almonds under broiler for 3 to 4 minutes.
Serve tuna mix on rice and top with almonds.

Serves four.

TUNA QUICHE

1 egg and 3 egg whites
2 tbsp. flour
½ cup low-fat mayonnaise
½ cup non-fat milk
1 12-oz. can tuna, drained and flaked
¼ cup grated Parmesan cheese
⅓ cup diced scallions
1 9-inch frozen pie shell

Preheat oven to 350°. In a medium-size bowl beat eggs and mix in
flour, mayonnaise, and milk. Add tuna, Parmesan, and scallions and
mix thoroughly. Pour mixture into pie shell. Bake approximately 1
hour. Set out to cool slightly before serving.

This is good with a salad. It can be refrigerated after cooking and
reheated for lunch.

Serves two.

SWORDFISH WITH TOMATO SAUCE

1½ lbs. swordfish, about 1½ inch thick
1 tbsp. olive oil
1 16-oz. can puréed tomatoes with basil
1 tbsp. tomato paste
4–6 shallots, peeled and chopped
1 tsp. minced parsley
Dash salt and freshly ground black pepper
1 tbsp. lemon juice

Preheat broiler. Brush swordfish with oil and place in a shallow baking pan or dish that is also brushed with oil. Broil until lightly browned. Remove from broiler. Preheat oven to 400°. Combine tomato purée, tomato paste, shallots, parsley, salt, pepper, and lemon juice in a small bowl and pour over fish. Place in the oven and bake for 15 to 20 minutes until fish flakes easily with a fork. Serve.

Serves four.

SWORDFISH STEAKS

2 tsp. olive oil
¼ cup fresh lemon juice
2 cloves garlic, minced
1½ tbsp minced parsley
1 lb. swordfish steaks (about 1 inch thick)
2 tsp. capers

Mix oil, lemon juice, garlic, and parsley in a small bowl. Arrange swordfish in a shallow dish for marinating, then pour contents of bowl onto and around fish. Marinate for 30 minutes, covered, at room temperature. Preheat broiler or prepare grill. Grill fish for 9 to 10 minutes on foil that has an abundance of small holes created with a fork, or broil for 9 or 10 minutes. Remove and sprinkle with capers and additional lemon juice or lemon wedges placed on the side. This is great with steamed vegetables.

Serves four.

SCALLOPS WITH LEMON AND GARLIC

1 tsp. lemon juice
1 tbsp. cornstarch
2 tbsp. olive oil
2 cloves garlic, minced
2 tbsp. soy sauce
½ tsp. ginger root
1 8-oz. can sliced water chestnuts, drained
6 large scallions with 3 inches of green, cut
4–5 oz. snow peas, caps and strings removed
1¼ lb. bay scallops, rinsed and drained

In a small bowl mix lemon juice and cornstarch until thoroughly combined. Set aside. In a large non-stick skillet heat oil over medium-high heat, add garlic, soy sauce, and ginger, and cook for about 1 minute until garlic is just starting to brown. Stir in water chestnuts, scallions, and snow peas. Cover and steam for about 2 minutes, stirring frequently. Stir in scallops, cover, and cook for another 2 to 3 minutes, stirring once or twice. Mix lemon sauce again, add to scallops, and stir until thickened. Served with a salad, this makes a very healthy dinner!

Serves four.

FRIED RICE WITH SHRIMP

2 eggs
⅓ cup soy sauce

2 tbsp. dry sherry

⅛ tsp. freshly ground black pepper

2 tbsp. cooking oil

1 clove garlic, minced

1 tsp. grated ginger root

¼ cup chopped onion

3 cups cooked rice

1 cup peeled, cooked shrimp, halved lengthwise

1 cup canned peas

In a small bowl beat eggs, then add soy sauce, sherry, and pepper and mix. Preheat wok or large skillet over high heat; add oil. Stir-fry garlic and ginger in hot oil for 30 seconds. Add onion; stir-fry about 1 minute. Stir in rice, shrimp, and peas. Cook, stirring frequently, for 6 to 8 minutes. While stirring constantly, drizzle the egg mixture over the rice mixture. Cook, stirring constantly, till eggs are set. Serve. Keep cooking to a minimum to prevent veggies and shrimp from losing their nutritional value.

Serves four.

HALIBUT WITH SPINACH

1 10-oz. pkg. frozen chopped spinach

¼ tsp. ground nutmeg

4 cups water

⅓ cup lemon juice

1 small onion, sliced

¼ cup chopped celery

¼ tsp. salt

⅛ tsp. freshly ground black pepper

4 halibut steaks (about 1½ lbs. total)

¼ cup grated Parmesan cheese

Lemon wedges

Cook spinach according to directions on package. Drain well; stir in nutmeg. In a 10-inch skillet combine water, lemon juice, onion, celery, salt, and pepper. Simmer 5 minutes. Add fish; simmer, covered, 5 to 10 minutes or until fish flakes easily. Carefully remove fish to a medium-size baking dish or a broiler-proof platter. Spread spinach over each halibut steak. Sprinkle Parmesan atop each. Broil fish portions 4 to 5 inches from heat for 1 to 2 minutes. Garnish with lemon wedges.

Serves four.

Grilled Tuna

1 tbsp. minced garlic
2 tbsp. balsamic vinegar
1 tbsp. finely chopped basil
1 tbsp. finely chopped mint
3 tbsp. olive oil
1 tsp. sugar
Dash cayenne pepper
Dash salt and freshly ground black pepper
2 tuna steaks

Combine garlic, vinegar, basil, mint, 2 tablespoons oil, sugar, cayenne pepper, salt, and pepper in a small bowl and mix. In a small or medium skillet, or a grill pan, heat remaining oil to medium high. Brush mixture on tuna steaks and grill for 1 to 2 minutes each side. Serve with Herb-Grilled Vegetables (page 228).

Serves two.

Spaghetti Squash with Clam Sauce

1 medium spaghetti squash
1 12-oz. can minced clams, with juice
1 tbsp. olive oil

1 large onion, chopped fine
2 tsp. minced garlic
Dash freshly ground black pepper
⅓ cup minced parsley
1 tbsp. lemon juice

Cut squash in half. Microwave on high in a microwave-safe bowl for about 4 minutes to soften, one half at a time. Set aside to cool, then with a fork, "comb" the squash to produce long strands. Drain clam juice into a small bowl. Heat oil in a large skillet and sauté onion and garlic for 3 to 4 minutes on medium-high heat until tender, adding pepper to season. Add reserved clam juice and cook on medium heat until liquid is reduced somewhat—about 3 or 4 minutes. Add clams, parsley, and lemon juice during the last 2 minutes of cooking. Add squash strands to the skillet for 1 minute to heat. Take off heat and serve.

Serves four.

SUMMER RISOTTO

1 tbsp. olive oil
1 tbsp. low-salt butter
1 cup diced onion
1 cup cut green beans
½ cup chopped red bell pepper
½ cup diced carrots
2 cloves garlic, minced
1 tbsp. minced parsley plus extra (for garnish)
1 tbsp. chopped fresh basil
2 14-oz. cans vegetable broth or low-salt chicken broth
½ cup dry white wine
½ cup water
2 cups uncooked brown rice
4 tbsp. freshly grated Parmesan cheese
¼ tsp. freshly ground black pepper

Heat oil and butter in a large skillet over medium-high heat. Add onion, green beans, bell pepper, carrots, and garlic and sauté, then add parsley and basil. Put broth, wine, and water in a large saucepan on medium heat. Add rice and cook, stirring often until the liquid is nearly absorbed. Add vegetable mixture to broth and rice. Stir in Parmesan and pepper, and garnish with parsley.

Serves four.

Linguine with Clam Sauce

2 12-oz. cans chopped clams (reserve juice from 1 can)
1 cup non-fat ricotta cheese
1 tsp. olive oil
½ cup chopped onion
1 clove garlic, minced
½ cup dry white table wine
½ tsp. salt
½ tsp. (fresh or dried) basil leaves
Dash freshly ground black pepper
1 cup cooked linguine

In a blender container combine clam juice and ricotta and process until smooth; set aside. In a medium skillet heat oil over medium heat; add onion and garlic and sauté, stirring occasionally, until onion is softened, 1 to 2 minutes. Add ricotta mixture and wine to skillet; stir to combine. Reduce heat to low and let simmer 5 to 7 minutes, stirring frequently. Add clams, salt, basil, and pepper and let simmer until clams are heated through, about 1 minute longer. Serve clam sauce over hot linguine.

Serves two.

SEAFOOD LINGUINE

1 tbsp. olive oil
8 scallions, thinly sliced
3 cloves garlic, minced
½ lb. cooked, peeled, deveined medium shrimp
1 8-oz. can cooked crabmeat, picked over and flaked
2 tbsp. dry white wine
1 tbsp. lemon juice
¼ tsp. crushed red pepper flakes
¼ tsp. dried thyme
¼ tsp. salt
1 16-oz. box uncooked whole-wheat linguine

In a large non-stick skillet, heat oil and add scallions and garlic. Sauté, stirring constantly, about 2 to 3 minutes. Add shrimp, crab, wine, lemon juice, pepper flakes, thyme, and salt; cook, stirring constantly, until heated through, about 3 minutes. Cook linguine according to directions on box and serve topped with the seafood mixture. This is good with a light salad for dinner.

Serves four.

ZUCCHINI-RICE QUICHE

1½ cups cooked brown rice
1½ medium zucchini, shredded and drained
2 tbsp. canned chopped green chilis
1 cup shredded reduced-fat sharp Cheddar cheese
1 cup skim milk
2 eggs and 3 egg whites
¼ tsp. freshly ground black pepper

Preheat oven to 375°. Spray a nine-inch pie plate with non-stick cooking spray. With moistened hands, press rice evenly onto the bottom and up the sides of the pie plate. Top evenly with zucchini and chilis. In a medium bowl combine ½ cup Cheddar with milk, eggs, and pepper. Pour over the zucchini mixture; sprinkle evenly with remaining Cheddar. Bake until the top is golden and a knife inserted in the center comes out clean, about 45 minutes. Let stand 5 minutes and serve. This is a great healthy dish for afternoon or evening, and it's delicious reheated, too.

Serves four.

EGGPLANT PARMIGIANA

2 tsp. olive oil
½ cup chopped yellow onion
½ cup chopped green bell pepper
2 12-oz. cans puréed Italian tomatoes
¼ tsp. garlic powder
¼ tsp. salt
1 tsp. freshly ground black pepper
1 eggplant, pared and sliced crosswise
2 oz. grated Parmesan cheese
2 oz. shredded mozzarella cheese

Preheat oven to 400°. In a saucepan heat 1 teaspoon oil on medium heat, then cook onion and bell pepper for 1 to 2 minutes. Add tomatoes, garlic powder, salt, and pepper. Reduce heat and simmer, stirring occasionally until thickened. Brush eggplant slices with remaining oil, put on baking sheet, and bake for 10 minutes per side. Set aside. Put Parmesan in a shallow bowl and coat eggplant with Parmesan. In a casserole dish, spread one-third of the tomato mixture, top with one-third of the eggplant, and repeat sequence twice more. Sprinkle unused Parmesan and mozzarella on top. Bake 15 to 20 minutes and serve.

Serves four.

LIGHT DESSERTS

I don't often indulge in desserts, but there are, of course, occasions like holidays when a light dessert is in order. For this reason, I have included some of the ones I use. Cookies are probably the one treat I do have available for the kids, and I will occasionally have one or two in the middle of the day.

Taken in moderation, a dessert or a sweet is fine. The point I always stress is that eating foods that will put on weight must be kept to a minimum. And if you are exercising regularly, one or two cookies every now and then won't "weigh" on you. Personally, I believe that an occasional cookie will keep you feeling young and bring out the child in you. So enjoy a treat now and then and, by keeping your discipline, you will be happy and healthy. Remember: *Keep it smart and simple!*

SUNNY YOGURT

½ cup non-fat cottage cheese
⅓ cup skim milk
2 tbsp. sugar
1 tsp. lemon juice
⅛ tsp. ground cardamom
Few drops almond extract
½ cup plain yogurt
8 medium-size peaches

In blender container or a food processor bowl combine cottage cheese, milk, sugar, lemon juice, cardamom, and almond extract. Mix till smooth. Add yogurt and chill. At serving time, cut fresh peaches into wedges. Put in individual serving dishes and spoon sauce over peaches. Keep refrigerated for future servings.

Serves eight.

Banana Bread

2 cups all-purpose flour
1 tsp. baking powder
1 tsp. salt
½ tsp. baking soda
1 cup sugar
½ cup vegetable shortening
2 eggs
¼ cup low-fat sour cream
1 tbsp. lemon juice
1 cup mashed ripe bananas
1 cup chopped pecans
¼ cup wheat germ

Preheat oven to 350°. Grease a baking pan. Sift flour, baking powder, salt, and baking soda into a medium-size bowl. In a large mixing bowl mix sugar and shortening. Add eggs, sour cream, and lemon juice and beat well. Mix in mashed bananas and stir in pecans and wheat germ. Add flour mixture and stir to combine. Pour into the baking pan and bake 50 to 60 minutes until golden brown and a knife stuck in the center comes out clean. Cool before serving.

Pumpkin Pie

1½ cups pumpkin purée
2 tbsp. butter
¼ cup sugar
1½ tbsp. pumpkin-pie spice
¾ cup evaporated milk
2 egg yolks
4 egg whites
1 9-inch unbaked ready-made pie crust

Preheat oven to 350°. In a large bowl combine pumpkin, butter, sugar, pumpkin-pie spice, evaporated milk, and egg yolks and beat well until blended thoroughly. Set aside. In a separate bowl beat egg whites. Gently stir them into the pumpkin mixture. Pour filling into crust and bake for 50 minutes or until a knife or tester comes out of the pie clean. Let cool for a few minutes before serving.

CARROT CAKE

2 eggs and 2 egg whites
3 tbsp. packed brown sugar
1 tbsp. vegetable oil
1 tsp. vanilla extract
1⅓ cups instant non-fat dry milk powder
¾ cup whole-wheat flour
2 tsp. baking soda
2 tsp. ground cinnamon
3 cups grated carrots
1 cup canned crushed pineapple (no sugar added)
¼ cup dark raisins

Preheat oven to 350°. Spray baking pan with non-stick cooking spray and set aside. Using electric mixer in a medium bowl, mix together eggs, sugar, oil, and vanilla until mixture is light and fluffy; then, at low speed, mix in milk powder, flour, baking soda, and cinnamon, until thoroughly combined. Add remaining ingredients and stir to combine. Pour batter into pan and bake 40 to 45 minutes (until a cake tester comes out clean). Let cake cool for 5 minutes before removing from pan. Cool for 15 minutes before serving.

OATMEAL COOKIES

½ cup all-purpose flour
¼ cup sugar
½ tsp. baking soda
1 tsp. baking powder
¼ tsp. salt

¼ cup packed brown sugar
¼ cup low-fat margarine, softened
1 egg
2 tbsp. plain non-fat yogurt
¼ tsp. vanilla extract
1 cup quick-cooking rolled oats

Preheat oven to 375°. In a bowl mix together flour, granulated sugar, baking soda, baking powder, and salt. Add brown sugar, margarine, egg, yogurt, and vanilla; beat well. Stir in oats and chill for 2 hours. Drop by tablespoons onto a greased cookie sheet. Bake about 8 minutes. *Time saver*: Go to your local market and pick up some low-fat oatmeal cookies. Use the extra time to take a walk. Also, occasionally have a cookie as a nice afternoon snack.

Makes about 2 dozen cookies.

ALMOND COOKIES

¾ cup whole almonds
5 tbsp. low-salt butter or margarine
1 cup brown sugar
½ cup sugar
1 egg
1 tsp. vanilla extract
1 tsp. almond extract
¾ cup whole-wheat flour
1 tsp. cinnamon
1 tsp. baking soda
3½ cups old-fashioned rolled oats
8 oz. crushed pineapple
1 cup raisins

Broil almonds on a baking sheet for about 4 minutes, turning after 2 minutes. Take out, let cool, chop, and set aside. Combine butter or margarine, brown sugar, and granulated sugar in a bowl and mix well.

Add egg and vanilla and almond extracts and beat. In a separate bowl mix flour, cinnamon, and baking soda, and add to first mixture, stirring in. Add oats, pineapple, raisins, and almonds and mix well. Spoon small portions onto cookie sheet and bake at 350° for about 10 minutes until lightly browned. This is one sweet item I do enjoy occasionally.

Makes about 2 dozen cookies.

OATMEAL-RAISIN COOKIES

1 cup all-purpose flour
1 cup uncooked old-fashioned oats
1 tsp. salt
½ tsp. baking soda
¼ tsp. ground cinnamon
½ cup packed dark brown sugar
½ cup frozen concentrated apple juice (no sugar added), thawed
¼ cup vegetable oil
1 tsp. vanilla extract
¾ cup dark raisins
2 egg whites
⅛ tsp. cream of tartar

Preheat oven to 375°. In a medium mixing bowl, combine flour, oats, salt, baking soda, and cinnamon; set aside. Using an electric mixer, in a small mixing bowl beat together sugar, juice, oil, and vanilla; add to oat mixture and mix well. Stir in raisins and set aside. In a separate medium mixing bowl beat egg whites at low speed until foamy; add cream of tartar and continue beating until soft peaks form. Fold beaten whites into oatmeal mixture. Spray non-stick cookie sheet; drop batter by tablespoons onto sheet. Bake 10 to 12 minutes.

Makes about 2 dozen cookies.

Lemon Ice

2 cups sugar
4 cups water
2 cups fresh lemon juice

In a large saucepan, bring sugar and 2 cups of water to a boil, reduce heat, and stir continuously for about 5 minutes. Set aside to cool. In a bowl combine remaining water with lemon juice. Stir into syrup mixture and put into freezer for 1 to 2 hours. Transfer to a blender and blend thoroughly. Pour into a container and put back into freezer overnight. Let the ice sit out until slightly soft before serving.

Serves six.

Angel Food Cake

1¾ cups egg whites
1½ tsp. cream of tartar
¼ tsp. salt
1½ cups sugar
1½ cups flour
2 tsp. vanilla extract
¾ tsp. almond extract
¾ tsp. fresh lemon juice

Preheat oven to 350°. Beat together egg whites, cream of tartar, and salt in a large bowl until egg whites form soft peaks. Gradually add sugar, mixing at a lower speed, then add flour gradually, then vanilla and almond extracts and lemon juice. Transfer to an angel-food cake pan. Bake 45 to 50 minutes until golden. Take out and invert pan, letting cool. Put on serving dish. A nice light dessert.

Grocery List

This list is a basic guide. There are other healthy items you may want to incorporate into your diet. These are my staples and favorites. Learn what your favorite healthy food items are and begin adding them to your diet.

FRUITS

Cantaloupe
Honeydew
Oranges
Apples
Kiwis
Peaches
Strawberries
Mandarin oranges
Pineapple
Bananas
Papaya
Grapes
Blackberries

VEGETABLES

Mushrooms
Onions, yellow & red
Tomatoes, Roma & cherry
Romaine lettuce
Spinach, frozen or fresh
Peppers, green or red
Broccoli
Zucchini
Green beans
Carrots
Bagged/washed lettuce
Mann's Broccoli Slaw

DAIRY PRODUCTS

Non-fat milk
Low-fat Lorraine Swiss cheese
Low-fat Cheddar cheese
Eggs
Low-fat or non-fat yogurt
Low-fat Parmesan cheese
Low-fat or no-fat ricotta cheese

STARCHES
Brown rice
Potatoes
Pastas, whole-wheat
Bread & bagels, whole-wheat

SNACKS
Starburst
Gum (sugar-free)
Light popcorn
Oatmeal cookies

LIQUIDS
Tea bags
Bottled water
Diet soft drinks
(if you must!)

CEREALS
Oatmeal & rolled oats
Cream of Wheat
Bran cereal

SUPPLEMENTS
Women's One-A-Day
Wheat germ

MEATS AND PROTEINS
Shrimp
Scallops
Beans
Deli lunch meats
  (turkey, roast
  chicken, and other
  98 percent fat-free
  meats)

Turkey
Skinless chicken breast
Crabmeat
Extra-lean ground
  beef
Revival soy protein
  powder

Beef tenderloin
Fish
Pork tenderloin
Gardenburger
  veggie patties

SPICES AND DRESSINGS
Ginger
Balsamic vinegar
Sugar, brown & white
Chives
Spice blends (I like the
  Key West flavor)

Basil
Salt
Cider vinegar
Extra-virgin olive oil
Low-calorie, low-fat
  salad dressings

Whole pepper
Tarragon
Oregano
Parsley
Cilantro

Resources

AUDIO SUPPORT

Take It off with Julia series available at www.WeightLossByJulia.com

VIDEO SUPPORT

Master Charlie Foxman's *Powertone*, www.blackbeltedge.com
Tammy Lee's *Buns of Steel*, *Arms of Steel*, and *Abs of Steel*
Jennifer Kries's *The Method, Pilates Precision Toning*

NUTRITIONAL SUPPORT

eDiets.com

EXERCISE AND SELF-HELP BOOKS

Kathy Smith's Lift Weights to Lose Weight
The Four Agreements, Don Miguel Ruiz
Yoga, Rodney Lee
Over the Top, Zig Ziglar

MAGAZINES

Shape
Self
Cooking Light

SUPPLEMENTS

HGH: "Liquid Longevity." To learn more go to
www.longevitylabs.com.
Grow Young with HGH, Ronald Klatz, M.D.
Soy: www.revivalsoy.com/juliahavey

WATER FILTRATION

Brita

REWARDS SUPPORT

www.WeightLossByJulia.com
Weight loss motivation ribbon—www.ramseygems.com

Final Words

A few last words: 1) If you can use fresh, do so; 2) Don't make cooking or eating your focus; 3) Find twelve to fifteen recipes you like and use them frequently; 4) Exercise is a must for good health and can erase any extra calories you may take in; 5) Due to the compromised quality of food sources today, I recommend supplementing your intake with vitamins and minerals; 6) With almost every meal I drink water, although I have included tea as a suggestion or low-fat milk in the morning. I believe that getting enough water is the foundation of good health. If you carry a twelve-ounce bottle of water with you all the time, you will be making a big difference in your health.

Now that you know my story, you can use my experience to realize your dreams just as I have realized mine. Please visit me at my Web site, www.WeightLossByJulia.com, and let me know how you are doing and if there is anything I can do to assist you further. There you can learn how to join me for on-line chats, read success stories, submit your success story, receive additional motivational materials, or meet new friends who are on the path of Self-Improvement through Self-Motivation.

You do not need to journey alone anymore!

You can write to me at:

Julia Havey
P.O. Box 6794
St. Louis, MO 63144
Web site: www.WeightLossByJulia.com

Index